Toward a Theory of Child-Centered Psychodynamic Family Treatment

Toward a Theory of Child-Centered Psychodynamic Family Treatment: The Anna Ornstein Reader offers a clear introduction to Anna Ornstein's ground-breaking work on psychoanalytic child orientated family therapy. Drawing on her writing from across her long career and including new material, the book sets out her important theoretical work on the mind, self, development, and parental influences, and the therapeutic consequences of these concepts.

Anna Ornstein's self-psychological work is unique and outstanding. First published in 1974, a time when attachment and affect regulation theory had just started, Ornstein's work has developed far-reaching ideas, therapeutic concepts, and practicable approaches for psychodynamic children and adolescence therapy, based on the concept of analytic self-psychology, which has anticipated very early results of later affect regulation and attachment research. This kind of treatment considers parental work not as only accompanying, but as central, representing the core of the treatment process. The parental maturation process is directly described, which should enable the parents to accompany their child empathically, and therefore attachment-security enhancing. This treatment concept integrates the later findings of neurobiologically-based attachment and affect regulation theory which emphasizes that intrapsychic and interpersonal experience are in a continuous and everlasting exchange. In this book, Eva Rass offers a better understanding of Ornstein's approach, an insight into her life and work, and an introduction into the concept of analytic self psychology, followed by a selection of Ornstein's significant publications, in which the central concern is clearly elaborated, to give the reader a thorough introduction and understanding of her work.

This book will be of great value and interest to professionals working with children and families in psychoanalytic settings, and to students training in child psychoanalysis, psychotherapy, and family therapy.

Anna Ornstein, M.D. is a Professor Emerita of Child Psychology at the University of Cincinnati and a Lecturer on Psychiatry at Harvard Medical School.

Eva Rass is a psychotherapist in private practice in Buchen, Germany.

Toward a Theory of Child-Centered Psychodynamic Family Treatment

The Anna Ornstein Reader

Anna Ornstein
Edited by Eva Rass

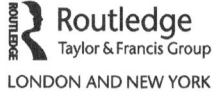
Routledge
Taylor & Francis Group

LONDON AND NEW YORK

First published 2021
by Routledge
2 Park Square, Milton Park, Abingdon, Oxon OX14 4RN

and by Routledge
52 Vanderbilt Avenue, New York, NY 10017

Routledge is an imprint of the Taylor & Francis Group, an informa business

© 2021 Anna Ornstein

© 2021 selection and editorial matter, Eva Rass

The right of Anna Ornstein to be identified as author of this work has
been asserted by her in accordance with sections 77 and 78 of the
Copyright, Designs and Patents Act 1988.

The right of Eva Rass to be identified as the author of the editorial
matter, has been asserted by her in accordance with sections 77 and 78
of the Copyright, Designs and Patents Act 1988.

All rights reserved. No part of this book may be reprinted or
reproduced or utilized in any form or by any electronic, mechanical,
or other means, now known or hereafter invented, including
photocopying and recording, or in any information storage or retrieval
system, without permission in writing from the publishers.

Trademark notice: Product or corporate names may be trademarks or
registered trademarks, and are used only for identification and
explanation without intent to infringe.

British Library Cataloguing-in-Publication Data
A catalogue record for this book is available from the British Library

Library of Congress Cataloging-in-Publication Data
Names: Ornstein, Anna, 1927– author. | Rass, Eva, 1947– editor.
Title: Toward a theory of child-centered psychodynamic family
treatment : the Anna Ornstein reader / Anna Ornstein ; edited by Eva
Rass.
Description: Milton Park, Abingdon, Oxon ; New York, NY :
Routledge, 2020. | Includes bibliographical references and index. |
Identifiers: LCCN 2020006771 (print) | LCCN 2020006772 (ebook) |
ISBN 9780367439408 (hardback) | ISBN 9780367439385 (paperback) |
ISBN 9781003006572 (ebook)
Subjects: LCSH: Child psychotherapy. | Family psychotherapy.
Classification: LCC RJ504 .O75 2020 (print) | LCC RJ504 (ebook) |
DDC 618.92/8914–dc23
LC record available at https://lccn.loc.gov/2020006771
LC ebook record available at https://lccn.loc.gov/2020006772

ISBN: 978-0-367-43940-8 (hbk)
ISBN: 978-0-367-43938-5 (pbk)
ISBN: 978-1-003-00657-2 (ebk)

Typeset in Bembo
by Wearset Ltd, Boldon, Tyne and Wear

Contents

1 Introduction

Eva Rass

Due to her pioneering work, Anna Freud was the most influential person in the development of psychoanalytic psychotherapy with children. During her lifetime, and even after, she influenced the scientific theory as well as practical aspects of psychoanalysis. Her work ranged from establishing psychoanalytic techniques in the counseling process with children and adults to the psychoanalytic application in educational and other psychosocial areas where she achieved outstanding results through fundamentally expanding the psychoanalytic theory (especially in the field of child rearing). She ensured efficient dissemination to various professionals in other fields of social work (Stumm et al. 2005, p. 159). Her concept of a psychological development line opened up the field of assessment to new areas and possibilities for evaluating a healthy child development. Overall, Anna Freud did her work in the area of psychoanalytic research and teaching with great sovereignty – both by writings and speeches.

Approximately 50 years after Anna Freud's classical work *Introduction to the Techniques of Child Analysis* (Freud, A. 1927), Anna Ornstein's paper *Making Contact with the Inner World of the Child: Toward a Theory of Psychoanalytic Psychotherapy with Children* (1976) was published. This scientific essay is based on the psychoanalytic concept of self psychology introducing a paradigm shift in the field of psychoanalysis which also led to a crucial shift within the psychoanalytic child psychotherapy: the focal point of observations was not only the drive and associated outcomes but also defense mechanisms, as well as the unfolding of the self. A changed perspective on development led logically to change in the treatment model where, with creative courage, Anna Ornstein developed a concept of child psychotherapy based on analytic self psychology.

In the last 40 years Anna Ornstein and her husband have written many far reaching essays in the field of clinical theory based on analytic self psychology where they worked as co-authors and published papers individually. Joint publications on theoretical and practical approaches in adult treatment were collected in some volumes, however, there is no comprehensive collection of scientific writings and publications in child psychotherapy. With one exception (Ornstein, A./Ornstein, P. 1985) Anna Ornstein published her "children essays" individually. However, the collection in this booklet does not portray the full spectrum of Anna's work. After reflecting with Anna on all her publications, we decided to integrate the most significant papers in this book. All writings were published between 1996 and 2012.

In order to understand the life and work of Anna Ornstein, the second chapter will portray an overview of her exceptional and unique way of life. A fundamental understanding and introduction into analytic self psychology by Heinz Kohut is needed as a base to proof and explain the theory and concept of child psychotherapy (Chapter 3).

Anna's work is characterized by her extraordinary courage to think critically in her own way, investigating concepts from recognized analytic child therapists that were seen as untouchable. In this context (Chapter 7) she rethought the case study of "Little Hans" based on a self psychological perspective leaving her with completely different results than S. Freud did during his lifetime. These results are so outstanding because the case study of "Little Hans" represents a fundamental building block for the Freudian concept.

Chapters 4, 8, and 9 will outline various main foci of theoretical and practical approaches by giving insight into A. Ornstein's concept of child centered family treatment. There will be focus on specific problems during the process of maturation classified by case studies. Tirelessly she sheds light on the developing child within its dynamic family bonding network, integrating Winnicott's concept that emphasizes parents' support to eliminate obstacles from appearing that adversely affect the developmental process of the child. The parental work in treatment is therefore not an accompanying process but rather a central procedure as the parents are the crucial mediators who have to continue the development of the child, even after therapy has ended. The co-authored essay with Paul Ornstein entitled: "Parenting as a Function of the Adult Self: A Psychoanalytic Developmental Perspective" describes the parental maturation process with the aim of enhancing the caretaker's perception of the child's experience and needs to provide conditions in everyday life important for growth in a sensitive, empathetic, and secure environment (Chapter 5).

Chapter 10 describes the fate of the "Children of Theresienstadt" who survived traumatizing life situations without any attachment to parents but with an existential attachment to each other. After being rescued, these children were brought to England where they lived in an orphanage with caregivers being supervised by Anna Freud. The adult lives of these children were based on emotional responsibility that opens up perspectives in attachment experiences between children. *Love Despite Hate* is the title of the book describing the unique fates of these children (Moskowitz 1983).

Chapter 6 discusses the fate of two young adolescences, Anne and Vivienne. The main focus will be on the environment of both girls and the importance of idealized adults who should support a healthy upbringing especially with view of major deficits in the early development of the self. Both girls left unusual writings of their unique experiences. In Vivienne's case, Anna Ornstein worked out the causing factors of suicide and analyzed through "telescopic" psychological work the early deficits in the development of the self which were not successfully "reorganized" during early adolescence.

Due to analytic self psychology perspective on babies – not as a drove bundle that solely discharges its tensions, seeking bliss in a joyful nirvana – infants are realized as actively striving for mutual reciprocity and engagement with the environment. Therefore, self psychology could easily integrate findings from infant observation studies and attachment, and affect regulation research into its concept. Long before infant/toddler-parent treatment was conceptualized, Anna Ornstein developed the child centered family treatment using the central attachment based principals of empathy, regulation, and secure attachment.

In this respect, the first writing from 1976 is still scientifically up to date and acknowledged. Through regulation, responsiveness, and empathy parents can develop the much needed attachment security and it is therefore necessary to take the primary caregivers as co-therapists. The therapist functions as a mediator helping the parents to approach and to experience the psychological misery of the child with the goal of initiating change and therapeutic progress. In order to achieve real structural changes this process represents the main focus of therapy.

The essays collected in this book encompass early childhood up until early adolescence: the children from Theresienstadt; case studies of school aged children; the fates of two female teenagers; and the 15 year old Tommy who had fallen into great despair. He had lost his father and was not able to find a comfortable place in his family. Based on theoretical observations, both the positive development of the self and its failing can be well comprehended. The self psychological concept of human development leaves no doubt that child therapy can only be performed in the interplay between therapist, child, and parents – stressing the importance of parents within the child's treatment.

References

Freud, A. (1927): *Einführung in die Technik der Kinderanalyse.* Leipzig/Wien (Internationaler psychoanalytischer Verlag).

Moskowitz, S. (1983): *Love Despite Hate, Child Survivors of the Holocaust and Their Adult Lives.* New York (Schocken Books).

Ornstein, A. (1976): *Making Contact with the Inner World of the Child. Toward a Theory of Psychoanalytic Psychotherapy with Children.* Comprehensive Psychiatry 17, New York (Grune and Stratton).

Ornstein, A.; Ornstein, P. (1985): Parenting as a function of the adult self: A psychoanalytic developmental perspective. In: Anthony, J.; Pollock, G. (Ed.): *Parental Influences in Health and Disease.* Boston (Little Brown and Company).

Stumm, G.; Spritz, A.; Gumhalter, P.; Nemeskeri, N.; Voracek, M. (Ed.) (2005): *Personenlexikon der Psychotherapie.* Wien/New York (Springer).

2 Insights in the life and work of Anna Ornstein

Eva Rass

Anna Ornstein was born on 27 January 1927 in Szendro (Hungary). She lived in her hometown until 1944 when she and her family were deported to Auschwitz after Nazi Germany occupied her country. Together with her mother, Anna survived several concentration camps while her older brothers as well as her father died in Auschwitz. Before the war, her family had lived according to traditional Jewish rules and her parents were strongly influenced by intellectual streams which were not only based in Budapest, but also in Vienna, Prague, and other German speaking cities.

Both older brothers who did not survive the concentration camps had immense influence on Anna's emotional development. A large part of her fighting nature evolved through her own motivation of keeping up with her brothers physically and mentally. Anna Ornstein described the Hungarian time as a contradiction; on the one hand everyday life was rather primitive but on the other hand she was raised in a family with intellectual ambition and dreams about a better future. As a Jewish girl she was not allowed to attend high school and it was not until the school year 1942/1943 that she was able to move into a Jewish high school in Debrecen.

The Debrecen school was a boys' school that started accepting girls due to the country's difficult political situation. Girls were only accepted if they could prove the completion of Latin, Algebra, and French courses as well as successfully pass an entrance exam. The continuous home schooling effort of Anna's mother bore fruit and the young and highly motivated Anna was allowed to start her high school education. This life did not continue for long as after approximately two years the German troops invaded Hungary in March 1944.

Jews were not allowed to use public transportation and were herded up into a ghetto within a few weeks (Ornstein, A. 2007a, p. 80). At the beginning of June, just when American forces arrived in Normandy, Anna and her entire family were deported to Auschwitz. While teenage Anna was holding onto her mother, her father and his elderly mother were the first to exit the train which is the last memory Anna has of both of them. Again it was the foresight of Anna's mother who recognized potentially fatal situations and acted appropriately to keep them both alive. The living conditions were horrendous and prisoners suffered from malnutrition, exhaustion, cold, and disease but both survived this excruciating time through the courage and bravery of Anna's mother (p. 84).

Nevertheless, even the longest war has its ending and on 8 May 1945 the Russian troops arrived at the concentration camp in the Czech city of Parschnitz where mother and daughter worked in an ammunition factory. The "liberation" in itself was the opening of the gates and the survivors were basically sent on their own way. They had to figure out their own way back home and had to find food and shelter which was an extremely risky process in postwar Europe. Anna and her mother reached train tracks that surprisingly marked the railway track to Zagreb leading to Budapest.

The controller cleared a wagon for the Hungarian women and gave them food and water until they arrived in Budapest during the summer of 1945. Soon the two received the devastating news that they were the only survivors of their family of five. Again, it was the life wisdom of Anna's mother who found work and employment. This new place of work was not only a way to make money and feed her daughter, but also exposed itself as a way of healing; Anna's mother became the director of an orphanage where 40 children arrived after their parents never returned from the war and concentration camps. Anna Ornstein restarted her education right where she was forced to end it before being deported and registered herself in the Jewish high school in Budapest. Again, she was very fortunate and the principal of this high school was the former principal of the boys' school in Debrecen that Anna attended. He was very happy to be reunited with his former student (pp. 86ff.).

After Anna's return to high school, something unexpected and wonderful happened: Paul Ornstein whom Anna had known before the German occupation and the same Paul who fell in love with teenage Anna when they first met, had heard in Klausenburg that someone had seen Anna alive. He started his love-driven search for Anna and found her in Budapest. The reunion was overwhelming for both. Paul Ornstein had escaped from a Ukrainian work camp and was hiding in the basement of the Swiss embassy for the final few months of the war. Anna and Paul got married in March 1946 and escaped to west Europe with the help of a Jewish underground organization. They both arrived in Heidelberg where they started studying medicine (Ornstein, A. 2007a, pp. 88ff.).

During their studies at the Medical College in Heidelberg (1947–1951), Anna and Paul had barely any contact with German students. Instead they were members of a Jewish student association where they formed affectionate and family-like relationships with other war survivors. With lots of gratitude, Anna remembers an outstanding man named Hermann Maas – a Catholic dean – who had been sent to a concentration camp due to his membership of an anti-nationalistic underground organization. The experiences in postwar Germany were mixed: Anna and Paul encountered many Germans with different political convictions helping them to avoid taking on a prejudiced attitude or developing a generalization for all Germans (p. 89).

Anna Ornstein soon became a medical doctor and started her career as a medical specialist. At that time, there was the opportunity to immigrate into the United States and Anna and Paul decided to take this chance. It was during her first year of becoming a consulting physician that Anna noticed that she was more interested in the emotional difficulties of her young patients rather than their physical problems. At that time, there was the opportunity at the University of Cincinnati to specialize in the area of children and adolescent psychiatry which, however, meant that Anna had to start training in general psychiatry first (p. 91). In 1953, Anna and Paul's first daughter was born and Anna succeeded in bringing her mother to America.

Michael Balint was one of the renowned psychoanalytic therapists who frequently visited the faculty of psychiatry in Cincinnati. The importance of early child development was a main focus at the time and additionally Balint introduced Anna and Paul to focal therapy that uses psychoanalytic principles during a short therapeutic time. Margaret Mead also visited the faculty frequently followed by Heinz Kohut who held lectures and discussion groups. Psychiatrists who wanted to become psychoanalysts had to fly for one hour to get to Chicago as there was no psychoanalytic institute in Cincinnati at that time.

First, Paul Ornstein completed the psychoanalytic training; Anna completed the training later because she had three children at this time; eleven year old Sharone, six year old Miriam, and four year old Rafael. The program in Chicago was a traditional psychoanalytic program working along traditional concepts with the main focus being on Freud's work and the Ego Psychology (ibid. p. 92). In retrospect Anna appreciated the strict program as she was accompanied by outstanding supervisors. Both Anna and Paul remembered it as a streak of luck in their professional career that they came into contact with Heinz Kohut and his concept of psychoanalytic self psychology. Anna and Paul Ornstein were part of the privileged circle that frequently met with Kohut to discuss the ideas developed by him. The intense co-working led to an enriching friendship. The theory building of Heinz Kohut, i.e., the development of analytic self psychology, entailed major advantages compared to traditional psychoanalytic theories (p. 93).

The orientation toward self psychology was especially valuable for Anna's work as a child psychotherapist as she was able to assess the relationship between the child's inner world and its emotional development – with a healthy or pathological outcome. In addition, the books and writings by the outstanding child psychoanalyst Donald Winnicott had great influence on Anna's therapeutic thinking.

Based on the fundamental meaning of the self-object concept for development, Anna published her first essay in 1976 introducing the principles of child centered family therapy entitled "Making contact with the inner life of a child." This outstanding paper, which is still relevant today, can be compared to an overture of a grandiose opera as it describes substantial elements of the scientific work that was published years later.

With the publication of this essay, a flow of creativity and inventiveness opened up, releasing an immense work of scientific writings and presentations.

In more than 70 publications, Anna Ornstein worked on the process of interpretation within psychoanalysis and psychoanalytic psychotherapy where she co-authored mostly with her husband. She also addressed the psychopathology of the child, as well as the therapy of children and families where the process of revealing after surviving extremely challenging situations and its mastery was thematized (Stumm et al. 2005, p. 347). Her own experiences during World War II awoke an interest to distinguish results of trauma in early childhood from trauma that was experienced during adulthood. All around the world, Anna gave more than 400 presentations and seminars, alone and together with her husband. Many of her writings were published in German psychoanalytic journals and magazines such as the essays also presented in this book: "Making Contact with the Inner World of the Child" (1985) and "Parenthood as a Function for the Adult Self" (1994).

Anna Ornstein is a member of numerous psychoanalytic organizations, she is the founding member of the *International Council for Psychoanalytic Self Psychology* and *the American Academy of Child and Adolescent Psychiatry*. She is also part of the editorial board of many reputable psychoanalytic journals. Anna received many awards and recognitions from psychiatric and psychoanalytic societies in America (Stumm et al. 2005, pp. 347/348). When Anna retired in 2000, her title at the University of Cincinnati Medical School was Associate Professor of Child and Youth Psychiatry. Right after, Anna and Paul moved to Boston in order to be in close proximity to their children and grandchildren. Anna and Paul Ornstein were welcomed with open arms into the scientific community in Boston and both of them taught at various psychoanalytic institutes and as lecturers at Harvard Medical School.

After their immigration to the USA, Germany was the country where both felt wholeheartedly welcome as they undertook many visits presenting and teaching supervision groups and workshops. Many deep friendships were established with German, Austrian, and Swiss colleagues leading to interest and adaptation of fundamental concepts of analytic self psychology in Europe (Ornstein, A. 2007a, p. 96).

The work in a psychiatric emergency ambulance at the University hospital in Cincinnati led to ongoing therapeutic challenges. Working in such a challenging environment where transitions and life changing events and continuous difficulties become clear day after day requires an ongoing personal maturation process of the therapist especially for his/her updated knowledge. Anna Ornstein has always successfully faced these challenges and wrote down her experiences – a very personal way of "self regulation."

Besides the papers in this book, there are more writings and publications with a view at developmental processes of children and adolescents. Based on Anna Ornstein's agreement various other writings were chosen and summarized with the following topics:

A talk in Denver (April 1991) was entitled *Special Problems in Parenting in Single and Reconstituted Families* and described the extraordinary challenge that parents have to face after separation, partner loss, and new relationships where parents and step parents have to adapt to altered life routines. Parents have to deal with affected children which is not in their usual repertoire of emotions. The appearing emotions barely fit into a previously structured self, leading to difficulties fostering an empathetic connection to the child.

Major challenges start to arise when a stable parenthood breaks apart through a divorce. The separation often leads to finding new partners and getting remarried where each partner brings their own children into the new marriage. The mastery of this transition requires the full spectrum of emotional resources that an adult him/herself needs for everyday life. A child's suffering which arises through the inevitable transitions of a divorce exhausts the parental resources – especially in regards to the empathic approach, i.e., these changes in life often deplete the emotional resources and availability of the parents. Therapy endeavors to not only acknowledge the inner difficulties of the child but also take into account the urgent needs of the adult (either being a single parent, re-married, or becoming a step parent). Adults often have to put aside their own needs and emotional challenges. Conducting a treatment without a "holding function" for the parents can easily lead to a perceived "superimpose" that impairs the maturation process negatively. This essay clearly demonstrates how helpful the concept of psychoanalytic self psychology is as it repeatedly tries to assess the psychological well being of the patients while facilitating the development of a therapeutic process.

In 1997, the *Handbook of Child and Adolescent Psychiatry* was published and included Anna Ornstein's essay "School Age Development from a Self Psychological Perspective". This paper outlines clearly the different psychodynamic approaches, such as the concept of Freud, and the Analytic Self Psychology of Heinz Kohut with their different assessments of early childhood. This different perspective leads subsequently to a changed view about school aged children leading to a shift in the therapeutic approach. Anna Ornstein brings out very clearly Freud's concepts of the latency phase – i.e., the overcoming of the Oedipus Complex – what consolidates in this concept a well functioning superego and defense mechanisms.

The child is forced to take on the developmental task of successfully balancing defense mechanisms and drive. As the girl does not have to develop castration anxieties the development of her superego is evolving differently as there is a lack of overcoming the Oedipus complex and this leads to more difficulties in moral development. Analytic self psychology, on the other hand, looks at the latency phase as a consolidation of the core self, especially when it comes to the regulation of self-esteem and moral development. Based on his clinical observations, Kohut concluded that in a normal development, parents react with joy and pride about the developmental progress of their child who does not have to experience guilt and fear. It is only if the parental empathetic resonance is missing that sexual impulses and destructive aggression appear in the child's behavior.

During early childhood, the toddler idealizes the caregiver due to his/her strength and omnipotence followed in the latent phase by admiration of the caregivers' values and ideals. This idealization can also be directed toward a teacher, sport coach, or other heroes. From an analytic self psychology perspective, the internalization of values and standards proceeds gradually to a non-traumatizing de-idealization of the caregiver. The internalized values are integrated into the developing psyche and represent the basis for the moral development.

The growth of self-coherence and the consolidation of the regulatory system of self-esteem are based on brain maturation where a transition from sensory motor intelligence toward formal operations can be observed. Therefore, a growth of efficacy and extended competency is given. It is crucial that the caring environment of the child reacts positively with pride and joy toward the child's growth in order to integrate the newly developed competencies and skills into stable elements of the child's psyche. At the beginning of school, a relatively complex self system should hopefully have been developed, putting the child in a position to successfully save the newly formed values and ideas during times of failure, criticsism, and disappointment.

This internal regulatory system is not fully stable yet when entering school years and still depends on the support from an empathetic and responsive environment. When the grandiose feelings of a young child are not sufficiently transformed the child is torn between irrational overestimations and feelings of inferiority. This phenomenon can be especially observed within group settings. At this age, the child is still fairly attached to their caregivers but is also actively looking for separation and a peer group where there is competition in many ways. In the peer group, feelings of success and loss occur and therefore these experiences can be compared to a training camp preparing for life. Group settings are therefore ideal opportunities to develop moral values but also to strengthen the personal identity. Self psychology does not see the process of identification as an answer to castration anxiety. The child is rather looking at the caregiver to playfully mirror their personality – also in regards to being male and female.

In her essay "Self-Pathology in Childhood: Developmental and Clinical Considerations" which Anna presented at a conference organized by the Menninger Foundation (28 February–7 March 1981) in Vail, Colorado, she clearly discusses the assessment of analytic self psychology to psychopathological appearances during childhood. She outlines the unsuccessful selfobject transferences (mirror transference/idealizing transference) that Kohut describes in his work. Anna Ornstein points out that based on age-approximate, mirroring reactions, the grandiose self can evolve into the psyche and construct the pole of the bipolar self – i.e., ambitions and goals. The second pole forms throughout the internalization of the functions of the idealized parents leading to internalizing ideals and goals (Chapter 3). In between these two poles innate talents and giftedness are embedded, which can under optimal conditions evolve through the emerging core self. An empty and worthless self on the other hand is not able to let these innate talents and gifts develop appropriately. Anna clearly distinguishes this approach from Freud's drive theory that delineate its theory of psychoneurosis along drive resistance considering the psyche as a closed system; environmental factors – except during very early childhood – will be more significant for forming structures (i.e., ego, superego).

From the perspective of analytic self psychology even with small children, and especially during the latency phase and adolescence, the failure of the transformation of the infantile narcissistic structures can clearly be observed – through a lack of vitality and liveliness. Further depression, a lack of a self-esteem, limited self confidence, lack of joy, vigor, and enthusiasm, no initiative toward future and future goals or expectations can be perceived. Gifted children are often not able to develop these talents and experience continuous feelings of emptiness and worthlessness. Based on three clinical case studies, from different phases of life, Anna describes this problematic phenomenon: (1) a preschool child, (2) a child in latency phase, and (3) a teenager. These three examples shed light on the therapist's possibility to clearly understand these developmental disorders based on the concept of analytic self psychology.

From the perspective of analytic self psychology, parental empathy is the sine qua non for the fulfillment of the parental selfobject functioning. It is therefore the goal for the parents to develop these competences, i.e., that their support is a building block of the child psychotherapy. These new abilities can not simply be "added onto" the pre-existing personalities of the parents they rather require a helpful guidance throughout the process. Parental selfobject functioning is an active function and has to be distinguished from the identification process. Eventually, a young girl can identify herself with her very feminine and attractive mother but at the same time the mother might not be able to empathize and reflect the internal experiences of the young daughter. It is therefore crucial that the therapist stabilizes the core self of the parents in order to help them develop a more mature parenthood that supports basically the therapeutic process.

During almost every child psychotherapy process, the act of playing or the play itself takes on a key role. Playing can be seen as a facilitating communication tool between the child and an adult. Additionally, the child can use play – comparable to the dream – to communicate internal experiences. However, there are also children who are not able to play, providing hints on the child's psychic state. And so it is no surprise that Anna Ornstein takes care of this important topic. During a conference on Play Therapy on 10 March 1984 in Boston she presented the paper "The Function of Play in the Process of Psychotherapy: A Contemporary Perspective" which was published shortly thereafter.

Anna Ornstein emphasizes the importance of play within every psychotherapeutic concept (psychoanalysis, behavioral therapy, as well as relational therapy). Through play, it can be easier for a child to regulate difficult affects, to cope with fear and anxiety, and to process retrospectively trauma-based experiences. In psychoanalysis, Anna Freud, Melanie Klein, and D. Winnicott have given play an important role as a crucial building block of therapy, even though their approach and contact were very different. Anna Freud and Melanie Klein described the process of verbalizing and the translation of the primary process into the secondary processes as very important and Klein even used this approach for children under the age of two.

The play performance of the child should be a mirror of the unconscious and Winnicott saw play as a highly creative process; the therapist should not focus so much on the content but rather on its spontaneity and excitement for the game experienced by the child. The interpretation of the process might interrupt or prevent the flow of the play and should be avoided. This clearly represented a contradiction to Anna Freud's and Melanie Klein's opinion.

Further, Erikson's work can be seen as a very important enrichment to the psychoanalytic theories of play. He mentioned that a sudden termination of the play – through an interpretation – can be associated with a non-attuned behavior of the therapist as playing represents an experiential and changing process that can easily be interrupted through talking. This kind of communication between the therapist and the child was of great importance for Melanie Klein whereas the importance of parent session was greatly reduced. Klein considered the transference relationship between therapist and child with the described intervention as most healing. Subsequently Anna Ornstein's discussions of her treatment concept of child centered family treatment contradicted the treatment techniques of Melanie Klein. As already mentioned, in previous work Anna emphasizes her being led by Winnicott's idea, that the child needs to be seen as a psychological open system that continuously reacts to interactions in their environment. Because the child is spending most of his time with his caregivers it is of key importance that they should empathically understand the internal and emotional state of the child. This process is crucial in order to master removing obstacles through new and improved family based environmental conditions and to introduce the process to progression. Ornstein cited Erikson who also saw the advantageous conditions of a therapy session as not so important, rather he recognized the extended time of the familiar influence as more significant.

Anna Ornstein emphasizes the importance of the child's play so that the therapist can receive insight in the inner world of a child regardless of whether the perceived feelings are conscious or unconscious. If the child includes the therapist into the play process, the therapist should try to match responsively to ease the surfacing of painful and conflicting material. If the therapist enters into the play process with their own ideas it can often lead to a game crash (likewise observed by Erikson). Play interruption and termination can lead to the child's experience that the therapy room is "another" unsafe place and it can take a long time up until the child builds trust again to resume the inner process.

In analytic child centered family treatment, play is seen more as a diagnostic than a therapeutic tool. However, it is important that the therapist "translates" the insight he/she gets through the play process to the parents in order to jointly find the source of the disturbed behavior. Further Anna Ornstein describes the child parent interaction as a form of self-selfobject unit (Chapter 3) – an interaction mode anchored in the theoretical concept of Kohut stressing the interactional aspect that is contradicting to monadic core principle of traditional psychoanalysis. The core of psychotherapeutic work consists in the growth of parental empathy – the most important developmental motor for a stable and self appreciating self. With support and regulation from the empathic therapist, the parents have to be led to their own vulnerabilities and insecurities. This process enables the parents to successfully approach the pain of the child.

The conversation between the therapist and parents does not only revolve around the disturbing behavior of the child but rather around the initial causes. Once the parents understand that the behavior serves to drown frustration, pain, and the feeling of helplessness and worthlessness, they may develop an empathic approach for the reorganization of the child's self. This kind of parental work emphasizes the interaction between parents and child as "focal," whereas other aspects from the adult life which are not influencing the symptoms of the child are left unattended. The therapist tries through translating to create an empathetic therapeutic milieu and the therapeutic play situation helps the child to approach their inner experience. Therefore, the therapist makes it possible for the child and their parents to perceive themselves not as "bad" and "deficient," and he is making efforts in removing developmental obstacles of which Winnicott has already spoken.

Anna Ornstein describes in her self-portrayal (2007a, p. 79) that she retrospectively recognizes that an expectation seemed to be written into her life plan where she either would have studied medicine, or she would have chosen another academic career. As both of Anna's brothers died during the Holocaust, she always had the feeling that she had to live her life for all three of them.

Anna Ornstein is not only a scientist and an unusually gifted therapist, she is also an author of prose – about memories to slavery and freeing (2001) and writings for Jewish Passover which she read to her family for more than 25 years. Every year, Anna told a new story about the past she had never told before. Her family and friends encouraged her to write all these stories down. In 2004, under the title *Das Apfelgehäuse*, these Holocaust memories of a young girl with etching from Stewart Goldman were published.

Looking at the amount of her practical work and the large extent of her scientific contributions, it indeed seems that Anna has been creative for three people (herself and her brothers) while living a fulfilled life. Despite the tremendous losses that Anna and Paul experienced, both of them achieved a deeply positive and affirmative attitude toward life which is reflected and condensed in their therapeutic conceptualization.

The orientation toward Balint's work and the collaboration with Kohut led to a concept assessing that every human being strives to realize internally anchored opportunities. The basic anthropological assumption of psychoanalytic self psychology differs from Freud's psychoanalysis, as analytic self psychology does not emphasize the guilty, but rather the tragic human being. While Freud thought about the central theme of contradiction between infant and culture that only can be dissolved through a "forced civilizing process" through sublimation and repression of the pleasure principle, Kohut on the other hand thought of an infant seeking an environment which has to be attuned with their needs (Ornstein and Ornstein 2001, p. 10). Thus, there is no contradiction between the ego and the world and therefore no unavoidable disease causing conflict. For Anna Ornstein, the approach to self psychology was especially valuable for her work with children. It helped her to assess the relationship between the child's inner world and their emotional development within the normal and pathological development.

The previously summarized essays as well as all the writings in this book show Anna Ornstein's practical and scientific proceeding based on analytic self psychology. Further publications relating to the psychopathology of the developing child and its treatment follow this path consequently. In cooperation with her husband, Anna worked out that analysis, deep psychological long term therapy, and focal therapy do not differ basically from each other. They move along a continuum based on the establishing of the therapeutic process and on a developmental oriented psychological treatment theory. In particular, the development of the focal therapy concept is relevant for the work with parents, as the severe burden between child and its parents find a therapeutic approach. The theory and praxis of an independent concept of psychotherapy with children/teenagers and their caregivers will be thoroughly elaborated in the following essays.

References

Ornstein, A. (2001): *Versklavung und Befreiung – Jüdische Schicksale aus Ungarn und zeitgemäße Pessachgeschichten*. Konstanz (Hartung-Gorre).

Ornstein, A. (2004): *Das Apfelgehäuse*. Gießen (Haland & Wirth im Psychosozial-Verlag).

Ornstein, A. (2007a): Den Traum meiner Eltern leben. In: Hermanns, L. (Ed): *Psychoanalyse in Selbstdarstellungen*. Vol. VI Frankfurt/M. (Brandes&Apsel).

Ornstein, A. (2007b): Roundtable Conversation of Child Survivors of the Holocaust. *Psychoanalytic Perspectives* 5, 5–12.

Ornstein, A.; Ornstein, P. (2001): *Empathie und Therapeutischer Dialog. Beiträge zur klinischen Praxis der psychoanalytischen Selbstpsychologie*. Ed. by H.-P. Hartmann, Gießen (Psychosozial).

Stumm, G.; Spritz, A.; Gumhalter, P.; Nemeskeri, N.; Voracek, M. (Ed.) (2005): *Personenlexikon der Psychotherapie*. Wien/New York (Springer).

3 Insight into the concept of Analytic Self Psychology

Eva Rass

The description of the professional career of Anna Ornstein within the previous chapters has clearly shown how deeply she was influenced by the self psychological concept of Heinz Kohut and the collaboration with her husband Paul and Kohut. In 1971, Heinz Kohut, who initially trained in neurology and later in psychoanalysis, published "The Analysis of the Self," in which he investigated the central role of the self within human existence. He described differentially and comprehensively an integrated theory of the development of the structure formation of the self, of the psychopathogenesis and psychotherapy of self-disorders. Many of Kohut's ideas led to an innovative departure from the mainstream of psychoanalysis and represented a creative extension of the Freudian theory. For the development of his new concept Kohut needed a circle of competent and equal colleagues who critically discussed his new theoretical and clinical ideas with him. Anna and Paul Ornstein belonged to this intimate circle and both were active and creative thinkers with a meaningful place within this group. After Kohut's death, Anna and Paul continued along this path and deepened their own research within the realm that was originally inspired by Kohut.

Anna Ornstein's essays in this book are based on this theory and it is therefore important to present the concept of Analytic Self Psychology as this enables an approach and an understanding of these writings. While Anna Freud (1895–1982) followed into her father's footsteps creating a child therapy in which the overcoming of the Oedipus Complex was the organizing principle for the psyche, Anna Ornstein developed a very different therapeutic process focusing the interaction of the child with its parents as the basis of Self Psychology.

Traditional psychoanalysis is a psychology of intrapsychic conflicts focusing on inborn biological factors – the so called "drives" – which are seen as the origin of any form of motivation. Analytic Self Psychology on the other hand focuses on the individual's intrapsychic experience too. However, environmental and relational influences are seen as imprinting and formative. In order to sustain and develop the self, regulatory and attuned reactions from an affectionate human being (described as "object") are needed. These selfobject reactions are seen as selfobject functions of the interactive other (Wolf et al. 1989, p. 6).

Perhaps Kohut's most original and outstanding intellectual contribution was the developmental construct of the selfobject. Indeed, self psychology is built upon the fundamental developmental principle that parents, with their mature psychological organization, serve as selfobject that perform critical regulatory functions for the infant who possesses an immature, incomplete psychological organization. Infants and toddlers are thus provided at non-verbal levels beneath conscious awareness with selfobject experiences that directly affect the vitalization and structural cohesion of the self (Schore 2003, p. 109).

The selfobject construct contains two important theoretical components. First, the concept of the mother-infant-pair as a selfobject-self-unit emphasizes that the early development is essentially seen as interdependence between the self and the objects within a system. Kohut's emphasis on the dyadic aspect of the unconscious communication shifted psychoanalysis from a solely intrapsychic to a more balanced intrapsychic-relational perspective. Second is the concept of regulation. In his developmental speculation Kohut stated that the infant's dyadic reciprocal regulatory transactions with the selfobject allow for the maintenance of his/her homeostatic equilibrium. Regulation thus occupies the intellectual core of Kohut's model. The broad range of developmental and infant research as well as affect regulation and attachment theory confirm his approach to stress processing (Schore 2003, p. 110).

3.1 Self definition

The structured organization of experiences which enables a human being to feel a sense of self is often described as "the Self." This psychological structure can be experienced through a person's feeling of vitality, self-esteem, and comfort. The self develops and maintains under the condition that the environment actively engages as good selfobjects. The child is thus provided with selfobject experiences that directly affect the structural cohesion of the self (Kohut 1971, 1977).

3.2 Selfobject needs

To survive psychically, the infant needs an empathic and responsive environment which adapts to their wishes, needs, and tensions. If the child's psychic and physical balance is disturbed, the affective high tension states are usually grasped by the selfobject – mostly a familiar caregiver – who reacts in a soothing and caring way. The selfobject should have a mature inner organization that can comprehend the needs of the child appropriately, to then take the infant into their own inner organization in order to cease his/her homeostatic imbalance through empathic caring (Kohut 1971, 1977).

The first of the two steps is far more important for the child than the second, especially with regard to the developing abilities of a child to establish their own inner psychic structure through transmuting internalization – i.e., to consolidate a nuclear self. Thereby the immature psyche of a child participates in the mature psychological organization of the selfobject. This necessary two step sequence includes parental empathy and soothing physical contact which enables the child to merge with the highly developed psychic organization of the selfobject and the participation in the selfobject's experience of an affect signal instead of affect spread leading to a need-satisfying action (Kohut 1977, p. 87).

This sequence of tension regulation cannot be overestimated; if continuously experienced during childhood, the resulting stress processing system remains one of the pillars of mental health throughout life. In the reverse, if the selfobjects of childhood fail, then the resulting psychological deficits or distortions will remain a lifelong burden. If for instance, the selfobject overreacts hypochondriacally to the child's mild anxiety, then the merger with the selfobject will not produce the wholesome experience of mild anxiety changing into calmness, but, on the contrary will produce the noxious experiential sequence of mild anxiety changing into panic. The end-result in all these instances is a lack of tension-regulating structures. Furthermore it is important for the development of a cohesive self to make the useful experience of being effective, i.e., to influence actively the selfobject for satisfying needs. The pleasure and pride of influencing others plays a critical role for the consolidation of a stable self. It is also significant for the infant to realize that states of merger and bonding can actively be induced. Moreover the small child needs urgently to be mirrored, i.e., to be seen, validated, and admired: "Mum/Dad look at me" (in adult life this need exists too but in a more mature form). Seeing mother's and father's pleasure and pride in their child reflected in their eyes is an essential precondition for self-esteem and healthy self-confidence throughout life. Selfobject needs are existent in every stage of life. For infants, these selfobject needs are age-appropriate archaic, for adults they are modified and age-appropriate mature. If later in life these archaic forms emerge they may signal developmental arrests. To satisfy, selfobject must stand for a function, not a person. In a more mature state this function can be fulfilled through symbols, ideas, and real objects too.

3.3 The process of self-development[1]

The developmental moment where the infant or child starts to develop a feeling of having a self is difficult to define. It can be assumed that a newborn does not have a sense of self as described up to now. The biological rhythms of the unborn child are regulated by the physiological circuits of the mother. After cutting the umbilical cord, these rhythms need to be newly synchronized. After birth the mother no longer supplies the child through the umbilical cord but functions as an external coordinator of the child's biorhythms. Without these caring actions the child would not only starve or freeze to death but it would also die because of the chaos of the immature coordination of the physiological subsystems. Motor movements, arousal, sleep-wake and sucking rhythms, thermodynamic regulation, pulse, blood pressure, growth hormones, and neurotransmitters are all regulated through the mother's attuned caring accompanied by skin contact, movement rhythms, body warmth, smell, and periodic feeding.

The regulation of the inner physiological milieu of the child is therefore delegated to the interactions between mother and child. Only when the growing child has stored physiological experiences accompanied by affects in the cortex, can external stimuli be processed adequately internally. Therefore, in early life at a biological level, a selfobject is needed which fulfills life supporting demands, that the very early self is not able to complete on its own. If the selfobject is not able to provide the balance of these homeostasis needs which are indispensable for maturation then there is an increased risk for dysphoric states. In this context Winnicott speaks of "agonal fears" which will be imprinted deeply in the memory system without ever being put into words. These traces effects indelibly the affective core of a human being.

The infant requires a responsive empathic selfobject that provides them with the needed selfobject experience – i.e., mirroring (the glance from mother's eye) provides the fragile self stability and cohesion satisfying therefore the inborn need for vitality and confirmation for grandiosity, efficacy, and uniqueness. Merging with the idealized selfobject provides an experience of calmness and completeness. The main function of the selfobject should provide the developing self with the experience that it will be understood in its inner core – in the real inner self. This experience will provide the assurance of not being alone and being together with another self.

The healthy processes between the self and the object, the so called self-selfobject processes that build up a stable self, consist of two steps: first the empathic environment – the selfobject – is in synchrony with the psychological need-wishes of the child. Second, not traumatizing empathy failures from the selfobject must occur. Kohut called the result of such failures by the selfobject during childhood "optimal frustration." This two-step process, which happens frequently during early development, has important consequences. It leads to a structure building via transmuting internalization (1977, p. 87). This internalization is of great importance as it induces a process in which the child can build up their own stabilizing and tension-regulating structures for the maintenance of a more mature and cohesive self.

This mild deviation from the beneficial norm of the caregiver has to be endurable otherwise no transformation and therefore maturation can occur. The driving force for development is therefore the continuous search for inner equilibrium leading up to higher structural levels (Kohut 1977).

Presumably the infant has no idea of a "spiritual life"; such an idea might emerge around the eighteenth month of life. Through the sensitive affect attunement[2] (Stern 1985, pp. 138ff.) of the mother these perceptions of an inner life can only develop as she captures and mirrors the emotional states of her child. This allows the emergence of the child's feeling to be existent. The experience of psychic reality can only be achieved through shared experiences.

The psychomotor development allows the child to expand their activities in the second year of life. He/she begins to symbolize, to speak, and to play with thoughts. It is a great step away from the pre-verbal and intimate closeness into a world with different structures. The urge for independence and autonomy, the strong desire to complete things without help finishes the non-verbal delightful interaction between mother and child. A self concept develops and opens the possibility to perceive this self. By this time ontogenetically a monumental threshold will be surmounted; in phylogeny this developmental step took billions of years (Köhler 1995).

The expanded action radius leads to an elevated and festive mood. The words "No" and "Want to do it myself" are mainly used; this phase inevitably leads to collision with limit setting adults but also to the narcissistic injury as fine motor skills are not fully developed yet and the child is often disappointed when specific actions cannot be performed perfectly. The experiences of smallness, dependency, and deficiency can lead to "narcissistic rage" (Kohut 1971) because of their own failure. But this rage also increases the urge to one's own initiative and to explicitly do everything by oneself. Confrontations with caregivers will be tried. The selfobject has urgently conveyed to the child experience that this attitude is allowed and that after the collision the relationship with the caregiver is repaired.

The child is still fairly egocentric and is not able to imagine that others experience themselves differently than the child him/herself. The child in the sensorimotor phase lives in his or her own reality. It takes time to develop the ability to distinguish between phantasies, desire thoughts, and reality (Köhler 1995). During this pre-oedipal phase, a slow loss of the ideal parent-imago happens. Every imperfection that is noticed in the idealized parent leads to a corresponding internalization of the lost characteristics of the object. Parental strength is experienced by the child as a development-friendly gift especially when the parent reacts with an inner pride if the child has the courage to express his/her frustrations when wishes are not being granted.

These are "optimal" frustrations, that lead via internalization to structure building. The parental inability to say "no" can reflect that the child is phase appropriate developing an own self and is starting to separate from the parent's self and becoming independent. Sometimes the "loss" of the child is unbearable for the parents and they are not able to accept that a child is developing an independence. With every educational confrontation a minor external loss of the object is given. Every small loss in the external world of the child leads to an equivalent growth in his/her inner world – and becomes a sediment in the psyche of the child (Kohut 1979).

Selfobject experiences through mirroring, idealizing, aversion, efficacy, and "alter-ego"[3] are needed during the oedipal phase so that the developing self can adapt a gender identity. The strong, coherent, and harmonious self of the oedipal child becomes fragmented when his or her vitality comes across resistance. The unempathic parental reactions can happen through open and direct action or can manifest in defensive reactions or withdrawal. Under these conditions, the developing self of the child is prone to be fragmented and imbalanced, and his/her normal non-sexual affection and non-hostile assertiveness become sexual and hostile.

The same-sex parent will consciously or unconsciously realize that he or she has become the target of the rival aversion of the child reacting under favorable circumstances with self-esteem and empathically limit setting (Kohut 1979).

During pre-puberty phases, the various kinds of selfobject experiences expand. This often leads away from early caregivers toward teachers and friends. But especially their selfobject functioning can be substituted through symbolic substitutes. This beginning process will increase and deepen during adolescence. The cognitive development allows one to recognize the deficiencies of the parents with the result that these early selfobjects will be de-idealized. Because the self – which requires responsive selfobjects – cannot exist in this vacuum, the relationships to peer group members or admirable idols is so important. To master this severe developmental task other demands or expectations are pushed to the background (Wolf 1988).

3.4 Disturbing troubles and crisis in psychic development

Kohut was convinced that psychoanalysis will move away from the conspicuous incidents during childhood. There is no doubt that incidents such as birth, disease, and death of siblings; separation of families; long separations from important adults; or difficult and enduring disease of a child may all play important roles in the tissue of genetic factors often leading to psychopathology in later life. But based on clinical experience, it is mostly the psychopathological personalities of the parents, or of one parent, or certain pathogenic characteristics in the familiar atmosphere in which the child is growing up which are the cause for a failed development of unsolvable conflicts which characterize later adult personalities.

This means that it is not a single traumatic individual event that causes the child's failed development but it is the chronically failing selfobject environment leading to an easily vulnerable child and to an injured self. The important incidents during childhood might be seen to be the origins for later disorders and prove to be focal or turning points in memory. The occasional failure of the selfobject is not the course for a sickening and disturbing development but the chronic inability to react appropriately that in turn can be traced to psychopathology of the adult self (Kohut 1979).

The inability to achieve cohesion, strength, and balance in the self might be the origin for self-disorders, i.e., that the selfobject experience has not been sufficient. The self reacts and is vulnerable over the life span when the early childhood self experiences have been insufficient and inadequate. In early childhood the vulnerability is the greatest; but a self can be hurt at any age. Deficient interactions between child and the caregivers are experienced by the self as threatening or even damaging. Certainly there are differences in the genetic make-up but it is the reaction of the selfobject milieu to the innate deficiency that must be considered.

The developing pathology cannot necessarily be explained by an innate defect but rather based on the inability of the selfobject to react sensitively and adequately to a difficult situation. The ability of a parent to react empathically to the unusually big and specific selfobject need of such a child has far reaching consequences for the coherence of the growing self – even once it has become an adult self. Kohut (1977) describes the self as a bipolar

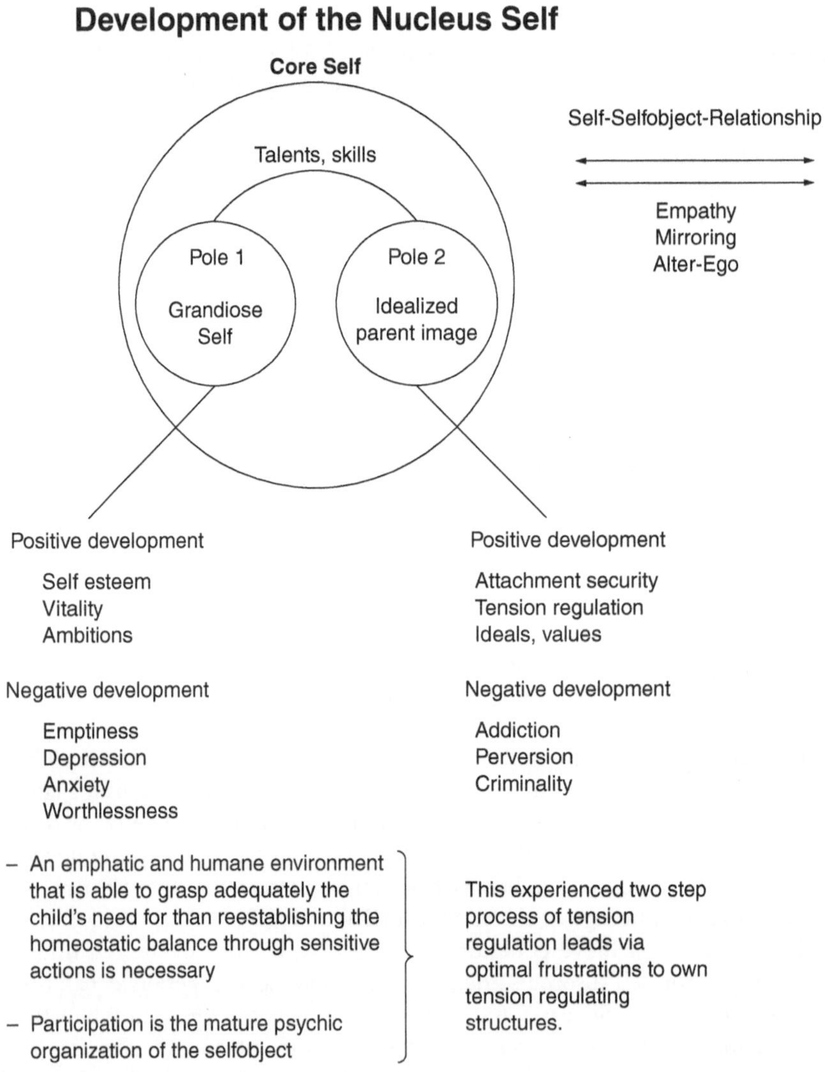

Development of the Nucleus Self

Core Self

Talents, skills

Self-Selfobject-Relationship

Pole 1

Grandiose
Self

Pole 2

Idealized
parent image

Empathy
Mirroring
Alter-Ego

Positive development

Self esteem
Vitality
Ambitions

Negative development

Emptiness
Depression
Anxiety
Worthlessness

Positive development

Attachment security
Tension regulation
Ideals, values

Negative development

Addiction
Perversion
Criminality

– An emphatic and humane environment
  that is able to grasp adequately the
  child's need for than reestablishing the
  homeostatic balance through sensitive
  actions is necessary

– Participation is the mature psychic
  organization of the selfobject

This experienced two step
process of tension
regulation leads via
optimal frustrations to own
tension regulating
structures.

Figure 3.1 Development of the nucleus self.

structure: One pole is formed through the mirroring selfobject experiences and the other is a pole of ambitions. The other pole evolves through the idealized selfobject experiences and is described as the pole of values and ideals.

The concept of analytic self psychology is based on a conciliatory co-existence between the self and the world. The environment cannot and should not be always perfect as it would adversely affect the healthy development. However the environment has to respond appropriately, empathetically, and adequately to the child's needs – in form of a selfobject milieu – so that the child has the chance to develop and consolidate a stable self-esteem. Over the lifespan this regulatory relationship plays a fundamental role for the maintenance, integrity, and vitality of a coherent self.

Notes

1 See Köhler, L. 1986/1995 in Rass 2002, pp. 128–132.
2 "Affect attunement" is the performance of behaviors that express the quality of feeling of a shared affect state without imitating the exact behavioral expression of the inner state ... Attunement behaviors recast the event and shift the focus of attention to what is behind the behavior, to the quality of feeling that is being shared (Stern 1985, p. 142).
3 Alter-ego selfobject experience: the object is experienced as being like the grandiose self or as being very similar to it (Kohut 1971, p. 115).

References

Köhler, L. (1986): Von der Biologie zur Phantasie. In: Stork, J. (Ed): *Zur Psychologie und Psychopathologie des Säuglings*. Stuttgart-Bad Cannstatt (problemata frommann-holzboog).

Köhler, L. (1995): Das Selbst im Säuglings- und Kleinkindalter. Vortrag beim 4. Internat. Selbstpsychologie Symposium (Dreieich), 15.–18.06.1995

Kohut, H. (1971): *The Analysis of the Self*. New York (Int. Univ. Press).

Kohut, H. (1977): *The Restoration of the Self*. New York (Int. Univ. Press).

Kohut, H. (1979): The two analyses of Mr. Z., *J. Psychoanal.*, 60, 3–27.

Rass, E. (2002): *Kindliches Erleben bei Wahrnehmungsproblemen*. Frankfurt/M. (Lang)

Schore, A. (2003): *Affect Regulation and the Repair of the Self*. New York/London (W.W. Norton).

Stern, D.N. (1985): *The Interpersonal World of the Infant*. New York (Basic Books).

Wolf, E. (1988): *Treating the Self. Elements of Clinical Self Psychology*. New York/London (The Guilford Press).

Wolf, E.; Ornstein, A.; Ornstein, P.; Lichtenberg, J.D., Kutter, P. (1989): *Selbstpsychologie. Weiterentwicklung nach Heinz Kohut*. Wien (Internationale Psychoanalyse).

4 Making contact with the inner world of the child

Anna Ornstein

4.1 Toward a theory of psychoanalytic psychotherapy with children

Psychoanalytic psychotherapy of children evolved out of the combination of psychoanalytic psychology, the direct observation of young children, and the study of the child's immediate and larger social environment, primarily the family and the school. The child guidance movement, a uniquely American approach to the treatment of emotional problems of children, remained carefully balanced between an emphasis on the child's inner life, on the one hand, and on the importance of the environment in the treatment of the child, on the other. The relatively heavy emphasis which most training centers placed on the individual treatment of children was primarily related to the influence of psychoanalytic theory on the practice of psychotherapy in this country. Anna Freud [1], with her pioneering work in child psychoanalysis, was the singularly most influential person in the development of psychoanalytic psychotherapy with children. This meant not only the application of psychoanalytic theory to the understanding of the child's psychopathology, but that the principles which guided the individual treatment of the child were also derived from psychoanalytic treatment principles. These principles, in turn, were to a greater or lesser degree similar to the ones employed in the analysis of adults. Though there are considerable variations regarding the rigidity with which the principles of analytic abstinence are being observed in child analysis, many child analysts maintain that children, no different from adults, can be treated by a focus upon their transferences, and that the only way to promote the analytic process with them is through the exclusive use of interpretations. Weiss takes issue with the practice of consulting with the parents on the same grounds as he does with giving the child candy or birthday gifts; namely that they all interfere with transference developments and detract the child from the work of the analysis. "If the child's pathology is in the past, if it is structuralized, then it can be analyzed within the transference. If the pathology is of the present and is a continuation of the past, that aspect which is current and not a transference onto the parents cannot be analyzed at that time. That which is transference, whether to analyst or to parent, can evolve into a therapeutic transference neurosis and is capable of being analyzed." [2].

The indiscriminate application of psychoanalytic treatment principles to children whose emotional difficulties were not the expression of internalized conflicts and their neurotic solutions, but rather related to structural defects and/or developmental arrests, led to considerable disappointment with the results of individual treatment of children. The theory of treatment in psychoanalysis in the early days of its application to child psychotherapy was still based on the theory of the psychoneuroses which it intended to "cure." The theory of psychopathology always determined the technical considerations employed in the treatment situation. Psychoanalysis has traditionally aimed at dealing with internalized psychoneuroses. The extension beyond the psychoneuroses to the character disorders and to developmental arrests or defects occurred subsequently. Thus, psychoanalytic psychotherapy does not have a theory of treatment of its own, as yet, neither in relation to adults nor in relation to children.

There are several reasons why a theory of treatment in psychoanalytic psychotherapy with children has never developed. First, there is the problem of the varied forms of psychopathology with which the child therapist is confronted. Children who fail to complete primary developmental tasks, both in terms of ego and superego development, manifest severe behavior disorders, narcissistic or psychotic symptomatology. These children only rarely establish a dependable therapeutic alliance or develop cohesive transferences which would make the primary or exclusive use of interpretations feasible in their treatment. With young children in particular, even when conflicts and their solutions are relatively well internalized, interpretations alone are of limited value. Increasing the child's awareness of the meaning of his behavior through clarifications and other forms of verbalizations is usually considered therapeutic. Joselyn, and more recently, Carek [3] maintain, however, that a child's improvement in treatment frequently cannot be traced to anything more specific than an "accepting relationship" or an "identification with the therapist."

The failure to develop a theory of treatment more specifically suited for psychotherapy resulted in the application of various trial-and-error techniques in the individual treatment of children. Certain aspects of psychoanalytic treatment principles were thus violated, while others were uncritically retained. For example, in psychoanalytic psychotherapy the parents are frequently consulted, and the child is actively wooed with gifts and other means, with the explanation that children otherwise would not establish a therapeutic alliance. Such measures, however, do not result in a therapeutic alliance as much as they may mislead the child about the purpose of his therapy. He may understand the gifts as rewards for his reluctant attendance. Actively creating a pleasant and friendly atmosphere is also supposed to help the child accept the pain of being confronted with the unacceptability of some of his behavior or features of his personality. The existence of a "pleasant atmosphere" which is being created with the help of candy and gifts, however, should not be mistaken for a functioning alliance. Therapeutic alliance means that the child is actively engaged with the therapist in a joint effort to understand the conflicted or the arrested aspects of his personality.

A further departure from psychoanalytic technique is related to the fact that interpretations of the child's behavior are not necessarily based on material which emerged in the therapist-child interaction but are rather based on information which the therapist obtained from the child's parents. Though such "interpretations" may be well-timed and given empathically, the child usually experiences them as painful criticisms which he will try to avoid by distracting the therapist into his favorite play activity or otherwise deny the importance of the therapist's comments. The therapist himself, fearful of losing the tenuously established rapport, finds himself making fewer and fewer comments which could potentially alienate the child. Therapy sessions, under these circumstances, tend to become play sessions without truly deepening the therapeutic engagement and enhancing the therapeutic process. Such play sessions, interspersed with so-called interpretations, are viewed as opportunities for the child to experience a nonjudgmental relationship with an adult and thereby foster healthy identifications. Joselyn's and Carek's observations that a child's improvement in treatment frequently cannot be traced to anything more specific than to an accepting relationship or an identification with the therapist appears, under such conditions, to be well-justified.

Does this mean, as it would appear from current trends, that there is no advantage in offering individual psychotherapy to a child who had developed emotional problems? I do not believe this to be the case. My own thinking about this question has strongly been influenced by Winnicott [4], whose approach to the treatment of children was primarily determined by developmental considerations. He was as mindful of the importance of the child's internal experiences (fantasies, conflicts. affects, and defenses) as he was of the role of the family in the treatment process. To this end, Winnicott recommended "the unblocking of the child's progressive maturational processes ... so that the change he had so achieved can be made use of by parents and those who are responsible in the immediate social setting."

How is the "unblocking" of the maturational processes to be accomplished? In Winnicott's 1- or 2-hour diagnostic-therapeutic interviews, the unblocking occurred through his unusual ability to make contact with the child in depth. The child's anxieties emerged through the drawings which he and the child produced together. This made in-depth interpretations possible without the child feeling exposed or caught, since he himself witnessed the emergence of the nature and origin of his fears and conflicts. Whenever therapist and patient are successful in making such joint discoveries, interpretations which communicate the therapist's understanding create bond which serves as the basis for further therapeutic work. This is the essence of a therapeutic alliance. Such in-depth interpretive response requires of the therapist the recognition of developmental factors, the nature of the defenses, the presence of structural conflicts, or structural defects as these are revealed either in the child's drawings or in his relatively scanty verbal productions. Winnicott possessed extraordinary diagnostic and therapeutic skills. Most child therapists need not 1 or 2 hours, but several months or maybe years to gain insight into the child's inner world. However, the task remains the same: the insights gained into the child's inner world have to be utilized not only in the therapist's interpretive responses to the child, but most importantly, they have to be made available to those in the child's environment who are primarily responsible for his or her emotional growth. Winnicott gave explicit directions to the parents as to their conduct and attitude toward the child. In his use of the "proper family setting" in the treatment of the child, he extended the concept of the "facilitating environment" to the treatment situation as well. This developmental approach was high-lighted by the fact that he remained in contact with the family for many years after his initial diagnostic-therapeutic interviews, carefully watching for possible upheavals at crucial developmental phases in the child's life. The limitation of this approach was not the degree of the child's illness, but rather that of the family setting: "There is a category of case(s) in which this kind of psychotherapeutic interview is to be avoided. I would not say that with very ill children it is not possible to do useful work. What I would say is that if the child goes away from the therapeutic consultation and returns to an abnormal family or social situation then there is no environmental provision of the kind that is needed and that I take for granted. I rely on the 'average expectable environment' to meet and make use of changes that have taken place."

Such ideal conditions as the "average expectable environment" rarely exist, and it remains the child therapist's primary task to create such "environmental provisions." In most families, such conditions cannot be taken for granted but have to be actively created. I find the concept of a therapeutic milieu helpful in this context, even though this has been associated with settings outside of the patient's home. The concept is helpful because it refers to the overall atmosphere, the total ambience of a setting which is deliberately created so that the patient's disordered behavior is not met with retaliation or provocation, but rather responded to with empathy which is based on the understanding of the unconscious roots of the child's behavior.

The therapeutic milieu on psychiatric wards and in residential treatment centers is created by mental health professionals. The effectiveness of the personnel not only depends on their understanding of the unconscious roots of the patient's unusual behavior but also on their ability to remain relatively free of mutually interlocking transference relationships,[1] emotional reactions which would interfere with their capacity to respond therapeutically to their patients in the most varied and, at times, difficult circumstances. But can a therapeutic milieu be created in the home where deep-seated and long-lasting emotional entanglements are likely to be responsible for the child's difficulties to begin with? Since, irrespective of the nature of the psychopathology, the child's difficulties frequently constitute an intrinsic aspect either of the whole family's interactional patterns or, more narrowly, of one or both parents' unconscious attitudes and conflicts, a preadolescent child cannot be treated without the family's participation. The child's psyche is a relatively open system, and therefore, the most decisive influences – not only pathological but therapeutic as well – must occur in his everyday interactions with his immediate emotional environment. Important daily events such as mealtimes, bedtime, and the child's relationship with his teacher, are the more obvious areas for the application of the concept of the therapeutic milieu. A therapeutic milieu in the home also means that the parents have to be helped to recognize the significance which minor events or casual verbal communications have on the child intrapsychically and how such communications (or lack of meaningful communications) perpetuate the symptomatic behavior.

But how are such changes to be effected in the environment short of long-term treatment? Creating a therapeutic milieu which is primarily responsive to the child's pathology limits the therapist's goals regarding changes he may otherwise consider of importance in certain members of the family. For example, a child's phobia may be intrinsicly related to the mother's separation problems but not to her sexual difficulties. A therapeutic milieu, short of treatment for every member of the family, can be created by focusing the therapist's efforts on the enhancement or creation of empathy in the parents toward the symptomatic child.

Gottschalk and his co-workers [5] have recently systematically investigated an open-ended group of parents with the explicit therapeutic aim "to increase the knowledge and use of the parents attitudes and behaviors that would achieve optimal growth and development of their children." In their follow-up study, they found that these child-centered parent treatment groups indeed produced a definite improvement both in the parents and in the children. A child-centered orientation to treatment means that after the therapist understood the unconscious meaning of the child's symptoms and behavior, he/she has to "translate" this to the parents in behavioral terms: Why this child is, at this time in his life, feeling or behaving in this particular way, and how is this linked to parental behavior and conscious and unconscious attitudes. By understanding such connections, the parents are enabled to mobilize their empathy toward the child.

Empathy is a function of the mind which enables a person to make a "temporary identification" with another person. Kohut [6, 7, 8], whose theoretical and clinical contributions to the problems of narcissism have most convincingly demonstrated that (1) empathy is an indispensable tool of observation of psychological phenomena and that (2) empathy is a powerful therapeutic tool, describes the latter function of empathy thus: "Empathy, the expansion of the self, to include the other, constitutes a powerful psychological bond between individuals which – more perhaps even than love, the expression and sublimation of sexual drive – counteracts man's destructiveness against his fellows. And, empathy, the accepting, confirming, and understanding human echo evoked·by the·self, is a psychological nutriment without which human life as we know it and cherish it could not be sustained." Christine Olden [9], in discussing adult empathy with children, makes the important point that some adults who do not have any difficulty in being empathic with young children, may not be able to do so with adolescents and that the reverse of this is true as well. In the case of young children, more than in the later phases of the child's development, the adult has to be able to abandon his secondary-process mode of thinking and appreciate the absolutes (black and white, good and bad) which are characteristic of the primary-process mode of thinking of the young child.

The most obvious block to parental empathy is the parents fear of reexperiencing their own childhood anxieties. When a child's sense of helplessness creates similar affects in the parent, the parent defends himself by becoming angry at the child for having exposed him/her to the sense of helplessness. Parents who have to maintain rigid and pathological defenses relative to their infantile affects, experience their children's development as a potential danger to their hard-earned repressions. Having been treated unempathically as children may also leave parents with a limited ability for empathy. A clinically frequent observation, and therefore worth a special note, is the situation where the difficulty one parent may have in being empathic with a child is compensated for by the other parent. When these children grow up to be parents themselves, they are particularly eager to be emotionally available to their children. Since they suffered from the lack of empathy by one of their parents, their own narcissistic vulnerabilities make them particularly attuned to their children's needs for mirroring or other forms of affirmation. They identify with their children's narcissistic needs rather than respond to them. Such situations are frequently described as "too much empathy," which is incorrect. These are also failures in parental empathy, since the parents' behavior is determined by their own, rather than the child's, narcissistic needs.

Putting the emphasis on the establishment of a therapeutic milieu in the home necessitates a reconsideration of the potentialities and the limitations of the individual treatment of the child. Instead of considering individual treatment as primarily responsible for changes in the child's pathology, it is more productive to view it as an ongoing diagnostic evaluation. This, then, is to provide the therapist with an in-depth insight to be utilized not only in his direct responses to the child (which are limited in their therapeutic effectiveness) but also as guidelines in the creation of a therapeutic milieu within the home.[2] [10].

It is the thesis of this paper that the translation of the child's intrapsychic experiences to the parents and to those who are responsible for the child's emotional development is primarily responsible for the creation of a therapeutic milieu and is therefore one of the most important aspects of the treatment of the preadolescent child. (The therapeutic milieu provides the preadolescent with the opportunity to complete developmental tasks and to undo developmental arrests. The adolescent who needs treatment may need a therapeutic milieu which facilitates (or at least does not interfere) with the adolescent's developmental task to disengage himself from his immediate emotional environment.) It is the translation of the child's symptoms and behavior into their intrapsychic meaning which can most successfully elicit the environment's participation in the treatment process, whether such participation consists of a brief consultation, periodic meetings with the parents, the treatment of the entire family, or only some of its members.

The following points will help in the elaboration of my thesis. (1) To the degree to which a child had internalized his conflicts and can develop transferences, he may be treated primarily by interpretations. However, even in these circumstances, it is essential to create a therapeutic atmosphere in the home which will not interfere with the child's treatment. (2) The more obviously the child's pathology is an expression of a developmental defect or a developmental arrest, the more dependent the therapist is on the utilization of a therapeutic milieu either within or outside of the home. (3) An essential aspect of the child therapist's work is his accurate assessment of the potentials and limits of parental participation in the child's treatment. The creation of the therapeutic milieu within the home will be limited by the degree to which the parents are able to develop empathy toward the symptomatic child. (4) Since children live in transferences with their own parents, even when parental attitudes toward the· child change in response to the family's treatment, the child may still have to be made available to the therapeutic impact of his environment. Changes in family patterns do not automatically assure changes in the child's pathology.

4.2 The effect of the theory of treatment on technical considerations

Those who continued to consider the child's intrapsychic experiences as essential in the child's treatment were left with the task of integrating the child's intrapsychic experiences with those or his emotional environment. Various techniques have been used to achieve this integration: (1) several members of the family would be treated individually and their treatment periodically correlated – the collaborative treatment method; (2) the symptomatic child would be seen jointly with one of the parents, usually the one who is either considered most intimately involved emotionally with the child or is more strongly motivated; (3) all members of the family would be seen jointly; and (4) a combination of all these approaches at different times in the treatment process.

Empirically, there appears to be good reason to believe that this kind of flexibility is of advantage. However, without a theory of treatment, the choice of a particular treatment method may be left to chance and be without rationale. Without an adequate degree of conceptualization as to why one may choose one technical approach over another, the therapeutic process which evolves in any one of these treatment modalities cannot be readily recognized. That is, without a theory of treatment, the process cannot be studied and improved upon, and it certainly cannot be adequately taught.

Before elaborating my own proposition for the development of a theory of treatment in psychoanalytic psychotherapy with children, I shall briefly discuss the problems related to two of the above mentioned techniques: namely, (1) the collaborative technique and (2) the family treatment technique.

4.2.1 *The collaborative technique*

Collaborative psychotherapy in which parents and child are treated individually and their treatment "harmonized" by the various therapists has been taught in most training centers but rarely used in the actual practice of child psychotherapy. It is worthy of note that in reviewing the literature on collaborative treatment, with limited exception (such as a case report by Krug and Stuart [11]), most of the contribution appeared in casework publications (Hallowitz [12], Hartman and Horn [13], and Szurek [14]). The technique of collaboration appears to be workable only if the members of the team do not add to the complexity by introducing their own professional rivalries and prejudices into the treatment process. It takes extraordinary skills and considerable time to coordinate the essential features of the manifest content when the unconscious meaning of such material has to be sorted out against the unconscious of more than one therapist. What we then witness rather frequently is that while some resolution of the original interpersonal conflicts within the family may occur, new ones develop which are related to the unconscious affects and attitudes of the various members of the collaborative team toward each other, as well as toward those members of the family who are not in their professional care. The therapeutic red thread is frequently lost under these circumstances, as various transference attitudes of the therapist intrude into the treatment process and complicate the resolution of the family's original problems. In addition, collaborative treatment may foster the family's expectations that the child's therapist will cure their child. To this end, parents bring in complaints relative to the child's behavior to their own therapists in order for this to be passed on to the child's therapist thereby inadvertently charging him/her with the responsibility "to do something with the kid." Such information, as I indicated earlier, rarely facilitates but frequently complicates the work of the child therapist. What is he to do? If he does not bring up the parental complaints with the child, he is not "doing treatment," if he does, he is confronting the child with information which the child himself had not volunteered to him. Should the therapist introduce the parental complaints, the child is likely to feel exposed and embarrassed in front of the therapist and feel betrayed by his parents.

Should collaborative treatment be chosen as the method because several members of the family need treatment, its success may be better assured if information flows from the opposite direction as well, that is, from the child's therapist to those of the parents. Since it is the child's therapist who can best appreciate the source of the child's anxieties and reasons for his symptoms and behavior, it is he/she whose insights into the child's inner world can be invaluable to the parents' therapists. As I mentioned earlier, the therapeutic milieu is built on these insights through which the parents are helped to recognize the relationship between the child's behavior and their own conscious and unconscious attitudes toward the child. Using the child's problems as the focus, the therapist can more specifically gear his treatment toward those aspects of the parents' personalities which may not be a source of difficulty to the parents themselves, but which significantly interlock, and therefore help maintain, the child's conflicts, or are (in addition to constitutional factors) responsible for the developmental arrest or defect in the child's personality. I shall later return to a more detailed description of the technique of translating the child's inner experiences to the parents and the problems related to this. At this point, I would like to turn my attention to the use of "family treatment" when the child is the presented patient.

4.2.2 The family treatment technique

Because the collaborative technique has proven cumbersome and has frequently failed in its most essential aspects, namely in the integration of the child's treatment with that of the parents, child therapists have turned more and more to seeing the whole family jointly, or at least those members who were most closely emotionally involved with the symptomatic child. But does this mean that the child therapist fosters the evolution of a family treatment process? For a family treatment process to evolve, the therapist's interpretive activities have to be directed to the interpersonal patterns within the family. Family therapists view the appearance of symptoms in any member of the family as an expression of a disorder in these· patterns. This may not be the child therapist's view of the genesis of the child's symptom. He may carry his theoretical bias, without his awareness, into the family treatment situation. Should he then focus interpretively on the overt clinical symptom and its meaning to the child personally, he may interfere with the evolution of a process which would facilitate the exploration, interpretation, and resolution of faulty interpersonal patterns in the family. There is a difference in the theoretical position, and therefore in the nature of the process which evolves when interpretations are directed toward the manifestations of the family's interactional patterns or when they are directed toward the symptomatic child. Not to keep these differing theoretical positions in mind may make the evolution of a treatment process[3] [15] impossible.

There is a reciprocal, dynamic relationship between the process of treatment and the content of interpretations: the therapeutic process evolves in response to interpretations and it is the hour-by-hour diagnosis of the process (the relative freedom of. communication among family members, the family's "use" of the therapist in family treatment, the presence or absence of a therapeutic alliance, the cohesiveness of transferences, or the degree of

working-through in individual treatment) which gives direction to the therapist's interpretive activities. To lose sight of one (the process) in this reciprocal, dynamic interaction is not to know how to proceed with the other
(interpretations). Under these circumstances, the child therapist may not have
a clear vision as to where he is heading. Is he heading or aiming toward the
resolution of the family's problems, or is he attempting to create a milieu in
which this particular symptomatic child can resume his arrested development
or resolve his conflicts? For a family therapist (even when he sees a patient
individually) to focus on the person with the symptoms would be to support
the family's pathological mechanism of adaptation by implicitly agreeing that
it is the individual rather than the family who is in need of treatment.
Whitaker [16], for example, maintains that focusing on subgroups, be this the
marital couple or one particular member of the family, "is a remnant of the
psychoanalytic intrapsychic mythology in that it denies the power of the total
family system." Bell [17] maintains a similar view stating that when "the
family comes to treatment, the difficulty with one of the children must be
accepted not as the symptom of an individual's disturbance, but as a symptom
of disrupted relationships in the family." In contrast to the collaborative treatment method, where the assumption is that where there is disturbed child
there is a disturbed parent, in family treatment the assumption is that where
there is a disturbed child there is a disturbed family. "Functionally, the child's
symptom is thought of as a· product of a disruption in family interaction, …
most usually a breakdown in intrafamily communication, and not as a product
of intrapsychic conflict."

   Viewing the family as a system in which each member carries out a certain
function in order to preserve the family's homoeostasis has been a theoretical
vantage point for most family therapists (Bowen [18], Bloch [19], and
Minuchin [20]). Technically, this means that no interpretations should be
offered which would not take the workings of the whole system into consideration. While systems theory constitutes an essential theoretical background in the field of family treatment, there are considerable variations as to
actual techniques used. For example, Bowen, a major proponent of systems
theory, radically departs from its technical consequences when, in a recent
paper, he puts the emphasis on the need for each family member to differentiate himself out of the family of origin. Instead of directing attention exclusively to the nuclear family's interactional patterns, he recommends that the
members of the family complete their developmental tasks of differentiation
within their family of origin in order to make the proper adjustment in their
current families. This is a striking recommendation; it appears to be the interpersonal counterpart to the emphasis which psychoanalysis places on the need
to work through the genetic precursors of current symptomatic behavior.
While psychoanalytic treatment offers an opportunity to recreate the genetic
precursors in the transference, Bowen recommends that patients with marital
and family problems return to their original family and actively engage their
family members in working out long-standing interpersonal difficulties.

"Any effort toward reducing the cut-off with the extended family will soften the intensity of the family problem, reduce the symptoms and make any kind of therapy far more productive. The essential message in this paper is to report on clinical efforts to completely by-pass problems in the nuclear family and to focus on working out relationships with the extended family." [18]. Jackson [21] and Satir [22] appear to stay technically closer to systems theory when they emphasize the importance of training the nuclear family in communication. ("Individuals learn to talk rather than live with each other." [23]). Whitaker [16], apparently the most conservative in his approach to family treatment, insists on the presence of all family members. If that is not possible, his frame of reference, and therefore his technical considerations, still remains oriented toward the family as a system, regardless of the members present at a. given treatment session. "The initial factor may be not so much a matter of who is there during the session, but where the therapist is at in his or her thinking, that is, the therapist's attitude toward what is going on and what it all means." [16].

I agree with Whitaker in his insistence that it is of crucial importance to maintain a theoretical frame of reference in conducting any kind of psychotherapy. There is no other way to follow and to foster the evolution of a therapeutic process. While the theoretical frame of reference is of the greatest importance relative to the evolution of the therapeutic process, it should be noted that the setting in which the treatment evolves also influences what may become available for therapeutic interventions. If the setting is that of a family therapy with all members present, what the individual members will reveal about themselves and how they will reveal it will be different from what may emerge either in a marital or in an individual treatment setting. This may be stating the obvious. However, in the context of this paper, it is important to keep in focus that when child therapists opt for family treatment they are dealing with psychological issues different from those which they would obtain in the individual treatment of the symptomatic child. Since the therapist's interpretive comments importantly affect the course that the treatment will take, a child therapist would have to choose (and then consistently maintain) a theoretical vantage point which is either child-focused or one which fosters the evolution of a family treatment process. A clinical example may clarify this point.[4]

A family of five had applied to the clinic with the primary complaint related to their 15-year-old son, Tommy. Tommy was insolent, refused to do the many chores around the family's farm which the other two children, 21-year-old John and 18-year-old Ellen, had quietly accepted as their duty. The children's father had died 6 year earlier. There had been a new father in the home for the last 2 years. Tommy's insolence and rebellious, angry behavior was disturbing every member of the family but, most importantly, John, who after his father's death, assumed primary responsibility for running the farm and holding the family together. His job was made difficult by the fact that while their mother drank heavily prior to the father's death, her alcoholism after his death had considerably increased. As Tommy said, this made him feel like he lost not one but both of his parents.

The treatment, which was conducted by a skilled family therapist, was videotaped for teaching purposes. One of the teaching exercises consisted of a child psychiatrist contrasting the theory of treatment which would be child-focused to the one which the family therapist had employed. The assumption was that the child therapist would use the same setting, the family treatment situation, but that her interpretations would be child-focused rather than directed to the family as a unit. As the process of the treatment on the video tape began to unfold, one could follow the family therapist's line of thinking and identify with her efforts to integrate the psychological profiles of each member into an interactional pattern which was unique for this particular family. Watching the therapist carefully eliciting information from each member, one felt as if she were sitting in the center of the family circle. She was obviously listening with a frame of reference which facilitated the processing of her data (the family's verbal and nonverbal communications) into a unique interactional pattern. In this process she had· to answer questions such as: Who does what to whom in this family? And how do the members of the family react to the verbal and nonverbal behavior of each other? Eventually, she had to determine where the primary dynamic weight was resting in this complex interactional pattern so that she could get a better therapeutic handle on it. It appeared that while she had given equal status to each member of the family, certain of them eventually emerged as being dynamically more "weighty" and therefore therapeutically more crucial than others.

The child therapist processed the data with a different frame of reference. Her vantage point was not equidistant from each member of the family; she was not sitting (conceptually speaking) in the middle of the circle, but on the same chair with her patient, angry and rebellious Tom. As a child therapist, she processed the family's verbal and nonverbal communications in terms of their likely effect upon this 15-year-old boy. She would have responded to the family in such a way as to facilitate a therapeutic process aimed at helping Tommy resolve his internal conflicts so that he too could utilize the good common sense and good will which the members of this family obviously had toward each other.

As the child therapist conceptually sat on Tommy's chair, she perceived the family's comments and expressions of emotions as if they were directed towards her, as if she were the rebellious and angry 15-year-old boy. She felt jealous of brother John for having mother look at him with love and appreciation – she could feel the jealousy particularly keenly when John began to sob uncontrollably as he spoke of the difficult times when their father died. She knew that Tom could not feel the sadness, he only felt angry and bewildered, after all, he was 9-years-old when their father died, and instead of feeling sad then he felt angry – angry at his father for dying and at his mother for drinking. This made her just as unavailable as if she had left him too. While unable to respond to the 9-year-old's anger, the mother turned for support to her older son. Over the years Tom's anger had been maintained as he witnessed a special relationship between his mother and brother – a relationship he could not have with either of his parents. His anger was continually acted out toward John by refusing his request to help around the farm.

The arrival of the new father only potentiated the boy's sense of isolation. Keeping the child's inner experiences in her mind, the child therapist had to remember the children's developmental position at the time of their father's death and how this may have effected their particular responses to the loss. She had to focus on the specific nature of Tom's anxiety (his unresolved grief, his jealousy of his brother, and a feeling of being totally unsupported by the others in the family) and the unique and special way in which he dealt with these affects, both adaptively and defensively. Similar to that of the family therapist, her theory of treatment also required an answer to the question "Who does what to whom in this family?," but with the primary aim of how Tom specifically had gotten caught up in the interactional patterns, one of which was the creation of a triangle between himself, his mother, and his brother. She was witnessing Tom's attempt to cope with his sadness and sense of isolation from the family by being sullen, angry, and rebellious.

I shall describe an exchange from the actual clinical situation to further clarify how a particular theoretical orientation effects the technical, that is, interpretive considerations. As John was bitterly complaining about not being able to reach Tom since he could not be made to feel guilty by scolding, the family therapist, noting John's frustration with his younger brother, said that John obviously very much wanted to be close to Tom and now seemed frustrated because Tom would not let him. This was an interpretation which intended to demonstrate a pattern of relating, namely, John's need to get closer to his brother and Tom's refusal to accept the gesture. Such an interpretation helps the family to become aware of the manner in which they relate to each other. Eventually the unconscious roots of these interactional patterns may then be uncovered, made conscious, and resolved. While the interpretation served the aims of the family therapist well, the child therapist felt that the comment may have left Tom feeling that he was not doing the "right thing" by not permitting his brother to get close to him and with this, feel further isolated.

The child therapist, with Tom in the focus of her thinking, would have said that John sounded puzzled by Tom's behavior and attitude. It seemed to her as if John needed help to figure out what caused Tom to be the way he was – so different from him and others in the family. Such a comment would have been intended to initiate a process which could have evolved into an understanding by the family of Tom's own reasons for being the way he was, namely, rebellious and angry. The child therapist would aim to elicit and foster empathy toward Tom so that by understanding him, the family would not have to continue to respond to his defensive sullenness but could help him face the sadness and the anger in himself.

The presence of a theory of treatment provides the rationale for the therapeutic moves by the therapist. The therapist's level and mode of activity is determined by the particular theoretical frame of reference which guides the content, the timing, and the wording of his interventions. The setting of a treatment situation (whether with the individual, the whole family, or only with one or two of its members present) effects the content of the material. The process which evolves, therefore, is effected by the setting as well as by the theoretical point of view. Both crucially influence the therapist's interpretive work.

4.3 Toward a conceptual integration of intrapsychic and interpersonal factors

In the first section of this paper I had discussed the importance of a therapeutic milieu in the child's treatment even in cases where the child had developed relatively well-internalized neurotic compromise formations. I had recommended that the child therapist should translate, in the clearest possible language, the unconscious meaning of the child's symptomatic behavior to those in his environment who are responsible for his further emotional growth, because such a translation facilitates the creation of a therapeutic milieu in the home. I consider this approach to the treatment of the preadolescent child a tentative answer to the now widely held view that a child's illness is as much an expression of intrapsychic compromise formations as it is the expression of the family's maladaptive interactional patterns. Not to recognize the former would· mean not to appreciate the presence of psychological structures (rudimentary as these may be) at any age in the child's life, and not to recognize the importance of the latter would be to assume that development is possible in an emotional vacuum.

There has been a shift in emphasis of the causation of pathology in children in the last 2 decades. Ackerman [23] notes that while 20 years ago the Child Development Center in New York, studying a series of families, moved conceptually from an emotionally disturbed preschool child to the dynamics of the family group, now 20 years later, has reversed the direction. Now, at the Family Institute (there occurred a change in the name of the institute as well), the study group is moving conceptually from "outside inward, that is, from the psychosocial evaluation of the whole family, back to its product, the child in the third generation." [23].

Though the Ackerman study had approached the relationship between the child and the family from both ends, from child to family and from family to child, the study has not yet provided "an adequate understanding of the border of the child's self and of the dynamics of interchange between self and the surrounding environment. Even to this day our conceptualization of such mechanisms as introjection and projection remains vague." [23]. What is known, however, is the fact that the relationship between child and family is reciprocal and interpenetrating; that it is not only the parent who effects the child but also the child who effects the parent. The parents' effect on the child, however, is developmentally and therapeutically the more crucial one. In this reciprocal and interpenetrating system, it is of great importance to differential between that which constitutes the "inner world" from that which is observable in interpersonal relationships. In the course of a child's life time, subtle forms of parental communications and unconscious attitudes may create long-lasting intrapsychic consequences in the child. Subsequent development of interpersonal patterns and ways of communication may serve the purpose to hide the areas of greatest vulnerabilities in all participants. These interpersonal patterns usually become new sources of anxiety which then again call for new internal compromise formations. Because of the complexity of this hierarchy of defensive structures, it may not be possible to work all of them through in the course of the child's treatment. The most expedient and the most meaningful way to reestablish contact between the child and his emotional environment is to enhance (or to create) parental empathy for the child's anxieties, conflicts, and narcissistic vulnerabilities.

Certain therapeutic settings may be better suited to learn about the child's (or the parent's) inner world, while others bring the interpersonal elements into better focus. The combination of individual interviews with periodic meetings with the family has proven to be a method which child psychiatrists employ with increasing frequency. This combination has the advantage that both parents and child are given the opportunity to discover aspects of themselves which they, because of years of failure in communication, cannot do in each other's presence. Family therapists look upon this practice with disdain since it is their primary aim to improve the family's system of communication and "keeping secrets" is greatly discouraged. However, for a child psychiatrist whose goal is to enhance or to create parental empathy toward the child, such an arrangement may best meet therapeutic goals. (In situations where the parent(s) is not capable of developing empathy toward the child, the child has to be helped to recognize such parental limitations.)

To demonstrate the importance of differentiating the interpersonal from the intrapsychic factors which makes an accurate translation of the child's inner world to the parents possible, I shall describe a brief clinical vignette. Evelyn was a 15-year-old girl. She was a quiet, rather shy child, attached to her mother but fearful of her distant and temperamental father. The family consulted the clinic when Evelyn became increasingly more irritable and moody. In several family diagnostic sessions, she remained quiet while her parents argued about one thing or another. The child would throw occasional, angry glances at her parents but say nothing. Eventually, she was seen individually where she again remained relatively silent. The therapist interpreted her silence as an expression of her repressed rage at her parents for fighting. The child, not knowing what exactly was disturbing her, said that the therapist might be right. She continued to see the therapist in individual sessions. In these, she described her despair about her looks, about her inability to think for herself, about not being able to make decisions, and being acutely uncomfortable in social situations. All her complaints were interpreted as being related to her rage at her parents· which she now had turned against herself. The therapist had actively encouraged the girl to express her disappointment in her parents in order to feel better about herself.

The therapist's preoccupation with the interpersonal aspects of the girl's behavior (her angry silences) did not permit him to realize that it was not repressed rage which caused Evelyn to be moody and withdrawn, but rather that she felt inadequate, that she felt defective in her personality and in her looks. If she was angry at her parents it was for their failure to see her depression. They admonished her for feeling bad about herself since they saw no realistic reason for that. She was a bright and pretty girl – weren't her worries foolish? When she asked for the individual hour, she had hoped her therapist would take her negative image of herself seriously. She was sent back to her parents to express anger. She was not sure she felt this anger and she could not meaningfully relate it to her defective self-image. This confused her and made her more resentful and withdrawn. In this case, as in many similar ones, the child therapist has the diagnostic task to recognize the nature of the child's internal experiences and not to stop short with the recognition and interpretation of the interpersonal patterns. The relationship between the two is more complex than to assume that interpersonal phenomena are simple externalizations of internal experiences. In this case the assumption was that the child's anger at her parents (manifest in the family interviews) was responsible for her defective self-image, rather than that this was due to a disturbance in the narcissistic cathexis of her body-mind self.

The technique of translating the meaning of the child's symptom in a manner which permits those in his environment to become therapeutic or to facilitate their therapeutic potential is a complex task. I shall first discuss the potentials and limitations of this approach, as far as the parents are concerned.

At the time when the parents sought or had accepted the recommendation for professional help, they had at least implicitly recognized that they had been caught in a neurotic web. Not understanding the nature, or rather the meaning of the child's behavior, they react to this with anger and disappointment. Such spontaneous, direct responses to the manifest behavior of the child create new problems which soon cover up or accentuate the original difficulties. Naturally, the parents do not act or respond to the sick child in unison (my references to "parents" in this paper is to refer to the child's emotional environment apart from the child's inner experiences). The three-way split which occurs when one of the parents allies himself with the sick child is frequently misinterpreted as the cause rather than the result of the child's difficulties. In evaluating the nature of the relationships within the family, one has to remember that parental attitudes toward their children change over the years, they become "layered" as it were, in response to the changes which take place in the child. The child's development is then effected by these changed attitudes, primarily because the environment is "out of step" with the child's emotional needs and has ceased to provide him with a "facilitating environment" which is the sine qua none for progressive emotional development. As I mentioned earlier, it is important to differentiate the interpersonal conflicts which have arisen between the child and his environment over the years and those parental attitudes which may have been originally involved in·the genesis of the child's pathology. The interpersonal conflicts presented at the time of the initial evaluation are usually the end products of years of pathological interactions. What appears to be particularly helpful at this initial phase is the therapist's appreciation of the parents' attempt to interrupt the downward spiral of increasing distance and antagonism between themselves and their troubled child by having sought professional help.

The parent's ability to become therapeutic may not have always been optimally utilized in the treatment of children. This is in large part due to a rather pervasive attitude among mental health professionals in which the parents are usually considered at fault, primarily for lacking sensitivity relative to their children's developmental needs. Anger and depreciation for having failed their children precludes any effort on the therapist's part to understand the reasons why the parents may not have been able to develop empathic capacities. The explanation for this can usually be found in the parents' own backgrounds. In addition to the parent's original difficulties to be in empathic tune with the child, the child's current difficulties create guilt, anger, and disappointment in the parent(s) which further interfere with whatever parental empathy may have otherwise been available.

To enhance the parents' therapeutic potentials does not mean to give recommendation as to how to interrupt or actively discourage the child's disturbing behavior. Particularly destructive are recommendations which ask for changed parental behavior without an appreciation for the parents' difficulty to comply; such recommendations are "grafted" onto the parents' pathology. Finding themselves unable to follow the therapist's recommendations, they become more guilty and less able to effect changes in themselves in relation to the child. A frequently occurring clinical example should make this point.

A young mother had regularly taken her 6-year-old son to bed with her after the sudden death of her husband. When the boy became enuretic she visited the clinic and was told that the boy had to get out of her bed – since this was the cause of his problem. The mother followed through on the recommendation which meant nightly tearful battles with the child. However, since her own affective state was not "treated," she could not remove him from her bed without ambivalence. The enuresis continued, and in addition, mother and son became increasingly more irritable with each other. As the mother's depression deepened, the child developed further symptoms; he had become provocative and inattentive at school. Since the mother's grief for her husband and need for closeness with the boy was not acknowledged when the recommendation to remove the boy from her bed was made, both of them experienced the separation from each other as intolerable.

From the point of view of the parents, the translation of the child's inner world has to take into consideration at least two important factors: (1) the parents' own intrapsychic reality, that is, their potential and their limitations to develop and maintain an empathic attitude toward the child and (2) the parents' ability to identify with the therapist's empathy toward the child's and their own current predicament. The initial interview with the parents, so frequently used to obtain the history of the child's development, is in reality, the parents' first therapeutic contact with the therapist. If the parents perceive the therapist's inquiries as attempts to find fault or to fix blame, the therapist will lose an important opportunity to help the parents utilize his empathy towards their own predicament as they make their first efforts to help their child.

In relationship to some parents, and certainly in a milieu which has been designed to be therapeutic, a successful translation of the child's intrapsychic experiences into behavioral terms may be all that is needed to change the course of events: instead of the negative spiral which had established itself when internal compromise formations were being continually reinforced by negative parental responses, the parents therapeutic attitude may, in a relatively brief period of time, help undo the interpersonal consequences of the original problems. Whether or not the child is able to utilize such changed parental attitudes depends on the degree of internalization of the original conflicts and their neurotic solutions. Individual treatment under these circumstances has the primary task to "reopen" the child's inner world and make it available to the environment's therapeutic impact.

I would like to illustrate with an example of how the in-depth understanding of a child's difficulties and its communication to the parents was all that was needed to prevent the development of a school phobia in a 12- year-old boy.

Martin had always been a good student, but now, in the sixth grade, just about to enter junior high school, his school work has rapidly deteriorated. He became sullen and withdrew from his family and friends as he became disturbed by his inability to do his school work. The parents, who were older than the parents of Martin's contemporaries, responded with a great deal of anxiety to the boy's difficulties in school. Their anxiety was not only the expression of their concern for the boy, but his withdrawal and failure to perform touched on their shaky selfesteem that Martin's good school record and pleasant personality had, up until now, been supporting. Martin perceived the source of the parents' anxiety and responded to it with further unconscious attempts to disengage himself from them. Because of his relatively strict superego and his basically appreciative attitude toward his parents, his was a passive attempt at disengagement. He did not rebel and did not feel angry but instead he "failed" in school, then felt guilty for disappointing his parents and withdrew from them. He eventually retreated from school altogether, remained at home where he tried to study but couldn't, and became increasingly more miserable.

In discussing Martin's situation with his parents, the therapist found that the parents had no difficulty in recognizing their inordinate emotional investment in Martin, which had, at the time of his approaching adolescence, become a burden to the boy. The parents' fear of their son's ultimate separation had made them increasingly more anxious and clinging. They had questioned him repeatedly about his friends and watched him more closely than most of the young people his age were being watched. Their relationship, which had always been good, did not change. Instead, Martin developed a symptom which – as neurotic symptoms do – served on the surface two contradictory but unconsciously compatible purposes. On the one hand, by failing in school he attempted to give expression to his separateness from his parents. On the other hand, the symptom expressed his own fear of separation, since not being able to progress in school kept him longer at home.

The expectation for him to continue to do well in school was well-founded on his performance so far. There was no increased pressure on him in this area which would have explained his difficulties. Rather it was Martin's perception of his parents' anxiety regarding his tentative attempts to separate from them which had interfered with his entrance into adolescence. The choice of the symptom was certainly not accidental. Performance in school was important to the parents because of their own lack of education and therefore was the most likely area for Martin to assert his separateness.

The consultation consisted of sharing this insight with the parents. Both parents were relieved by the fact that Martin's difficulties in school were not an expression of deep-seated pathology but rather that of a developmental need to disengage himself emotionally from them. The consultation was therapeutic as it did not question the parents' competence as parents. Their shaky self-esteem was not tampered with, nor were they made to feel guilty in the course of the interview. Instead of becoming defensive, which is almost always the case when parents feel guilty in relation to their child's difficulties, they appreciated the important role which they were to play in Martin's recovery. With the therapist's help, they felt that they could meet the challenge of helping Martin over this hurdle. Neither primary attention to the behavior (the lack of performance in school) nor an even slightly judgmental attitude towards the parents' inability to respond to their child's developmental need for separation and individuation could have helped to initiate a therapeutic engagement. In this case, as in others, the therapist was greatly supported in his efforts to translate the unconscious reasons for the child's behavior by the parents' genuine desire to help their child. The·parents' motivation in this is not different from the initial tentative motivation of any patient who wants to be relieved of suffering and psychic pain.

While on the side of the parents, the difficulty in the process of translation is related to the limits of their empathic capacity toward the symptomatic child, there are problems presented in the technique of translation related to the child as well. If the child is in treatment, the most obvious problem is related to the question of confidentiality. It is difficult for the child, at first, to see the benefits of the therapist's direct or indirect contacts with the parents. However, as the child's therapy progresses, it becomes part of the therapeutic work to help the child recognize those areas in his relationship with his parents where both his parents and he himself need the therapist's help.

Earlier in this paper, I referred to the frequently made clinical observation that interpretations alone are of limited value in the treatment of young children. Does this mean that children cannot achieve insight or that they cannot utilize it? Children are indeed capable of achieving insight, but there are relatively severe limitations set on their ability to utilize it; young children need their environment's help to·effect changes in themselves. In individual treatment, it is of considerable importance to help children recognize how their behavior may make it impossible for their parents to find out what they really want. Once the therapist understands and accepts the child's reasons for his behavior, the child will be able to appreciate better how his behavior may create an obstacle between his wishes and the parents' ability to meet them. He needs the parents to recognize the changes in himself and to affirm the legitimacy of his affects and wishes. It is for this reason that interpretations are of limited value; the insight which the child can gain through them has to be made use of by the environment as well as by the child.

The story of Amy will demonstrate this point: Amy was a 9-year-old girl. She had an older brother to whom she was very attached but who had recently become busy with his own activities and had been paying less attention to Amy. The brother, whose friend had psychotherapy some time ago, suggested to his parents that they consult with a child therapist because of Amy's frequent tantrums, her many fears, and her bedwetting. The parents were receptive to the idea; they had reached "the end of the rope" since Amy had become extremely controlling of them. She objected to just about everything the parents would do for her, the way they woke her in the morning, the kind of clothes her mother prepared for her to wear, and the manner in which they spoke to her. Both parents had extensive treatment experiences in the past. The initial plan was to see Amy individually and consult with the parents periodically.

After Amy had been in treatment for several months and had learned to trust the therapist, she spoke of her fear of dying, of her fear of abandonment, and of her fear that something would happen to her brother, toward whom she consciously only felt love. She was conscious of her ambivalence toward both of her parents but not toward her idealized brother. In her treatment she had· repeatedly described how unjustly treated she felt by her parents, situations which obviously were related to her need to test them and in which she felt they failed her. The therapist told Amy that her parents needed her help to understand her better, especially her feeling that they preferred her older brother and that she felt they didn't love her as much as they loved him. She agreed with this, but she was violently opposed to the therapist seeing the parents without her because after their initial interview, they had walked away from Amy while she was having a temper tantrum, saying that they were doing this on the therapists' recommendation. Amy was afraid that the therapist would again tell things to her parents which would make matters worse rather than better. She felt that her parents always managed to "turn things against me." The therapist understood her concern, and as their work together progressed, she told Amy that without the help of her parents, she would not be able to overcome many of the problems which they had between them, especially her conviction that she could never please her parents the way her brother did. The therapist asked the child if she would like to tell her parents how they could help her not to have temper tantrums and not to be so stubborn with them. The parents were invited to the treatment only at those times when it was fairly clear in the child's mind what she wanted to discuss with them. This was a slow process, but the experience proved to be therapeutically much more meaningful than if she had permitted the therapist to see her parents separately. It was of particular therapeutic benefit that in the joint hours, Amy also had a chance to learn about her parents' motivation for their behavior toward her.

Since the child had been describing situations in which her father would tease her and how this would infuriate her, Amy and the therapist decided to discuss this particular issue with the parents. In one of the joint sessions, the therapist offered a tentative interpretation to the father regarding his motivation to tease the child. The therapist said that the teasing seemed to occur at times when mother and daughter were at odds; could it be that teasing Amy was to make light of her behavior so that mother would cool off and not take Amy's stubborn behavior too seriously and thereby precipitate a fight? While the father was busy being a "lightening rod by teasing," he had not realized that Amy's conflictual relationship with her mother was too painful to her to be teased about. The interpretation led to many important insights. Amy was pleased that her parents had been helped to realize how painful these daily fights with her mother have been to her, that her contrary and stubborn behavior toward them gave her no pleasure but was the source of her many anxieties, and most importantly, that being contrary and stubborn with them was to test them in all possible ways because she felt that her parents loved her brother more than they loved her. Amy's testing created too many frictions and noisy interactions for her parents to hear the message behind them, which was that they prove their love for her. She told her parents she wanted her behavior to be taken seriously (and understood) since she didn't like these fights either. When her father teased her, she felt foolish and he made her only more angry.

This small, rather narrow segment of a lengthy therapeutic process was to demonstrate that the child's trust in the therapist does not have to be undermined by the therapist's communication with the parents as long as the child is aware of, or actively participates in, these communications.

The success of integrating the child's intrapsychic reality with the interpersonal experiences depends, to a great extent, on the care with which the child's therapist selects those features in the child's emotional environment which are most centrally related to the child's anxieties. The intrapsychic pathology of the parents, if not directly related to the child's, is not included in this conceptualization. The child's personality, special attributes, sibling position, or sex may activate in the parents some of their conflicts which would otherwise not become symptomatic. Similarly, the parents may have difficulties related to their work, marriage, or have other symptoms which are not directly related to the child's problem. For example, sexual difficulties interfere with the parents' own happiness, these, however, are usually unrelated to their ability to be responsive to their children's developmental needs. Though the current trend is to study child development from "outside-in," that is, to start with the environment and follow its impact on the child, when pathological interactions have to be reversed, it appears to be more effective and it requires less time to work from "inside-out," from child to parent. By focusing on the child's difficulties, it is possible to take a selective approach to the parents' total personality. It is this focus on the child which, I believe, is frequently lost in collaborative treatment, especially when in the course of treatment the parents become patients "in their own right." It is then that the important aspects of collaboration break down. In the process of what had become individual treatment of the parents, sight is lost of those special, for the parents not necessarily pathological, features of their personality, which most centrally interlock with the child's pathology. I shall use a clinical example to make my point.

A 10-year-old girl and her mother have been in collaborative treatment for 2 years. During this period, the mother was not helped to appreciate the source of the child's fears and the reasons for her clinging, demanding behavior. There has been no improvement, but rather an increase in this behavior and in the child's severe anxiety states and phobias. This was so, I believe, because the mother, not being aware of the source of the child's anxieties, could not adopt a therapeutic attitude towards her. The lack of improvement created additional frustrations in mother and child, resulting in considerable pressure on the child's therapist to "cure" the little girl.

Margaret was a very verbal, precocious, 10-year-old girl. Her parents divorced after an unhappy marriage when she was 3 years old. Her father moved to a distant part of the country and he visited the child only infrequently. The mother, a vivacious, attractive woman in her early thirties, began to keep company with eligible young men soon after her divorce. Margaret disliked most of these men but she reacted particularly adversely to the man her mother eventually married. Dick was a handsome, gregarious man, loud in speech and brisk in manner, whose enjoyment of life included the generous use of alcohol and a love for gambling. The mother was obviously very much attracted to this man and the child was slowly excluded from this new relationship. Since this made Margaret fearful of losing her mother, she became angry and demanding. The mother experienced the child's behavior as interference with her new-found happiness. Both because she felt guilty over distancing herself from Margaret and because Dick had repeatedly disappointed her by staying out late to drink and to gamble, the mother periodically would become very solicitous with the little girl and the two would then be close again, like in "the good old days." In addition to this unpredictable behavior on the mother's part, which was determined by her need for closeness and not by the child's, Dick too, was alternatingly seductive (he would engage in sexually-tinged teasing) and rejecting of the little girl. In the course of these events Margaret developed a severe case of obsessional neurosis and multiple phobias; she had to observe a series of rituals before she could go to sleep. Her fears and her rituals would be worse when her stepfather was at home and she could not fall asleep in her mother's bed. One of her most disturbing symptoms was particularly time-consuming but one which did not necessarily insure her of a restful night; she would still be frequently awakened with nightmares. The symptom was her need to tap her head at a certain spot in sets of threes, then in sets of twos, and then again in sets of threes. The counting would be endless and in itself would become anxiety producing. When, under these circumstances, she would try to contact her mother (usually with some excuse), the mother would understandably be irritable since she wanted to spend the evening with her husband. It was under these circumstances that the little girl would feel particularly lonely and anxious.

The mother, in her treatment, had given repeated examples of Margaret's attempts at controlling her at bedtime and her alternatingly giving in to the child and then becoming angry and irritable with her because she felt manipulated. Mother's therapist addressed herself to these neurotic interactional patterns and had repeatedly given the mother permission to feel entitled to her time and not to give in to Margaret's demands. The therapist felt that the child needed "limit setting" to help her accept the reality of her current situation with her new father in the home. The mother's attempts at limit setting, however, were not successful they increased the child's sense of isolation, made her only more anxious and demanding. Her phobias spread and the violence of her nightmares increased.

Throughout this treatment period the child's therapist had regular meetings with the mother's therapist, which did not mean that these meetings were "collaborative." The mother's therapist addressed herself primarily to the mother's attempts to free herself from the child's clinging and controlling behavior. The clinging, demanding behavior was understood only in interpersonal terms, and the caseworker's recommendations to set firm limits to the child were based on this level of understanding. The child's behavior was understood as being conscious attempts to control her mother, rather than the result of her being both sexually overstimulated and made to feel insecure in this new triangular situation. The limit setting was experienced by Margaret as a confirmation of her mother's rejection of her and as a retaliation for her anger and sexual arousal. This only increased her need to test her mother's love for her. Since the mother did not understand the child's anxieties and she experienced her behavior as personal attacks on herself, her own sense of helplessness increased which made her limit setting increasingly more punitive.

The child's therapist had a good understanding of the source of Margaret's fears and she used interpretations skillfully. These were usually directed at the child's anger at her mother, at her fear of retaliation, and at her fear of Dick who would playfully overpower Margaret when he was in· the mood to play with her and thereby overstimulate the child. However, the therapist could not at first see how the mother could help the child with these feelings. An incident prior to the little girl's first trip to visit her father helped the therapist to see the mother's potential therapeutic role. Margaret's symptoms became badly exacerbated with the upcoming trip to visit her father. Her nightmares now included visions of a burning airplane; she was sure she would die in an airplane crash. As the child became increasingly more agitated, she refused to go to bed to avoid her fears and the compulsion for counting had increased. At night she would anxiously wait for her mother to comfort her, while the mother and stepfather were planning their own summer vacation. When the child would become whiney and demanding, the parents, according to the instructions of the mother's therapist, ignored the child and periodically reminded her of her bedtime. In her therapy hour, the child spoke of her conviction that something dreadful would happen to her mother while she was gone and that if only her mother could have fun, she would be all right until Margaret returned. The child also described how excluded and lonely she felt when the two grown-ups continued their plan-making without atten-tion to her when she could not fall asleep the night before. The therapist interpreted to the child her anger at her mother for ignoring her and how this was responsible for her fears, both for the mother's as well as for her own safety while they were separated. She also interpreted the child's fear of being separated from the therapist, the only person who really knew how she felt. The child felt better after sharing her fears with the therapist, but there was no change in her continued preoccupation with burning airplanes and the many possible ways in which her mother could get hurt while she was away.

Why were these essentially correct interpretations not more effective? In discussing the case in supervision, the therapist – in response to previous dis-cussions relative to the mother's importance as a therapeutic agent – now "discovered" how the mother could be helped to deal more effectively with Margaret's demands for time and attention and at the same time, help to alle-viate her fears. Her discovery was that what Margaret wanted from her mother was not that she give up her time with Dick (she wanted her mother to have fun while she was away; she wanted her mother to be safe from her omnipotent wishes) but what she did want was an indication that her mother knew how Margaret felt. The child's therapist thought out loud; "If the mother knew that she was not responsible to make her little girl happy all the time, if she wouldn't feel so guilty for wanting some time to herself, she would not have to withdraw from the child. Then, instead of setting limits which never worked, she could let the child know that mother understood how excluded Margaret felt when she and Dick were planning a trip together." This discovery by the therapist was more meaningful than she had at first realized. It was the discovery of the therapeutic power of empathy. The mother need not give up her own life – this would most certainly further aggravate the child's condition, as it would be a response to her infantile omnipotence and not growth-promoting since it would not help her increase her sense of reality. The child needed her mother's help to accept the reality of her new life, primarily her frustrations, her anger, her sexual feelings, and her disappointment that she was no longer the only person mother cared about. Limit setting did not answer these questions; to the child these were done out of the adult's needs and were not responsive to hers. But the mother's recognition that the child felt left-out, angry, fearful, and insecure, and her acceptance of these feelings as being "legitimate" under the circumstances, had a greater therapeutic potential than when these feelings were only accepted and interpreted by the therapist.

Once the mother's treatment became oriented towards the child's difficulties, the therapist learned that the mother's inability to respond empathically to Margaret was not the function of her preoccupation with her new husband alone. Rather, Margaret's fears and obsessional preoccupations created anxieties, which severely blocked her empathic capacities: since her own mother was mentally ill, going insane was mother's worse concern. This resulted in her defensively distancing herself from the child's anxieties and obsessional preoccupations.

The mother's acceptance of the source of the child's fears, could no longer "wipe away" Margaret's bad feelings about herself for being demanding and angry. She continued to feel guilty for these archaic and intense affects. However, the modification of her superego, which was the task of her individual treatment, was more likely to occur once the mother could empathically accept these affects which were no longer acceptable to the child. Her individual treatment, giving her an opportunity to express her fears and anger more freely, had been extremely valuable to Margaret. Through the understanding and acceptance of Margaret's reasons for her clingy and demanding behavior, the mother could facilitate the resolution of the child's conflicts which, to a large degree, had by now become internalized.

A further statement on the question of limit setting seems in order. From this case example it would appear as if I did not consider the setting of limits to the child's behavior as being potentially therapeutic. In cases where the child's psychopathology is expressed primarily in angry outbursts toward the environment or is self-destructive, the firm response by an adult usually calms the agitated child. However, the child perceives the difference between firmness which is motivated to calm and to comfort him from that which is retaliatory in intent and he will respond accordingly. It is at moments like this that parental empathy may be the most severely taxed! "Giving in" to a child's unacceptable behavior expresses contempt rather than empathy toward the child and has severe consequences for later development. Guilt and self-contempt is then added to the child's already negative self-image which most: likely is the source of his aggressive, self-destructive behavior to begin with.

A brief description of a 7-year-old, severely acting out child, may serve as an example to demonstrate this point.

Johnny was a 7-year-old boy who had been expelled from second grade from several schools. His misbehavior included all known tricks, like sitting under the table, biting the teacher's arm, throwing pencils, and refusing to comply to just about anything that was expected of him.

Johnny's mother was a working woman. He was put in the care of a babysitter – who became an important and reliable person to him – at 4 months of age. His mother divorced Johnny's father in the second year of the boy's life, and he began to attend nursery school at age 2½. The mother remarried when Johnny was in the first grade. By then the boy had exhibited a rather severe behavior disorder which began when he first attended kindergarten. The new father tried to help Johnny by adopting a casual, pal-like attitude towards him. When, in the second grade, the mother sought professional help, she was advised that the boy's difficulties were related to her marriage and that marital therapy was the choice of treatment. Johnny was seen by a child therapist some months later after the parents discontinued marital treatment since they could not meaningfully connect their marital relationship to the child's difficulties. Johnny had introduced himself to the child therapist by first painting a picture of a burning house which burned down so furiously that it could not be saved. This was followed by a painting of a "monster" – a huge glob of black paint which he then tried to smear onto the therapist. The therapist, who commented on both of these pictures as Johnny's way of telling her how he felt about himself (filled with fury like the fire, hopeless in his rage, and feeling bad like a monster, all black inside), was successful in preventing the boy from smearing her with the black paint (which may have been his attempt to attribute badness to her in order to be able to tolerate his own). Johnny's first creative activity in the office was the making of a paper mache snake; an activity which made him obviously very proud of himself. When the therapist promised to keep the snake, the child tried to impress her how little he cared whether or not she would do so. On his return he searched the office with an eager gaze, insisting that he couldn't care less whether the snake was there or not. His activities in the office became frantic from here on; he wanted to make bigger and better animals, all the while insisting that they weren't any good and the therapist should feel free to discard them. Indeed, whenever he took one home, he would destroy it.

The child's tentative attempt to have the adults (therapist and his parents alike) respond to his creations – which were parts of himself – positively, filled him with anxiety. His narcissistic vulnerability did not allow the direct expression of the wish that the therapist keep his animals as valued parts of himself. He took some of the animals home in the hope that his parents would express their interest in him by saving the animals. When they failed him in this (unconscious) expectation, he destroyed his creations. They were bad, not deserving of their attention, the way he felt about himself whenever they failed to mirror him positively. Since he developed his behavior disorder early in his life, Johnny's self-esteem had completely eroded; none of the responses from his environment were positive, they contained only corrections and admonitions for his behavior which were continually reinforcing his monster image of himself.

Johnny continued to be a terror at home and at school in spite of the remarkable rapport he established with his therapist. His relationship with her was isolated from the rest of his life. The therapist's explanations of the meaning of Johnny's behavior to the teacher and to the parents brought to light the fact that almost all of Johnny's severe temper outbursts were precipitated by relatively small incidents which, however, had great importance to the boy. For example, whenever he was interrupted in doing his art work in school or whenever his mother did not look at him while he was speaking to her, he would become infuriated and have a tantrum. Parents and teacher, alike, felt that understanding these connections were not much help as long as they had to cope with his aggression and rage. Did understanding his behavior mean to give in to it? Obviously that would be the final blow to this boy's self-image. He needed his environment's protection and demonstration that they cared so they would not let him hurt himself and others. However, once his narcissistic vulnerability was appreciated by his environment, their therapeutic actions did not have to be restricted to setting limits to his temper outbursts and provocations, but could be employed toward healing the narcissistic defects in his personality. Setting limits is a palliative measure and as such, important in the overall treatment plan. The prevention of situations in which limit setting becomes necessary, addresses itself to the core of the pathology which, in this case, was related to the child's narcissistic vulnerability. His rapport with his therapist indicated that Johnny was not "closed" to his environment's therapeutic influence. Appreciating the child's cautious way in which he asked for recognition (through the paper mache animals), he was open for the kind of mirroring which could therapeutically meet his narcissistic needs.

4.4 Toward a theory of psychoanalytic psychotherapy with children

In this final section I shall attempt to evolve some general principles toward a theory of psychoanalytic psychotherapy. These principles will be based on the clinical observation that the enhancement or creation of parental empathy is central to the treatment of children and that this objective is best achieved when the meaning of the child's symptoms is translated into behavioral terms to his immediate emotional environment. In order to enunciate these general principles, the following clinical-theoretical framework should be kept in focus. (1) A developmental diagnosis of the child may be the best guide in deciding on the form of treatment (collaborative individual or family). (2) The integration of the intrapsychic with the interpersonal factors is a crucial aspect of the child therapist's work. Towards this goal, I propose that regardless of who is in treatment (only one or both parents, with the child being seen only diagnostically, the child in treatment with periodic consultations with the parents, or all members of the family in on-going treatment individually or jointly), the totality of the treatment be conceptualized as occurring in a single process. (3) The use of a model may be of particular value in processing the complex psychological data that are generated when several members of a family are in treatment. The model depicts visually the notion of the single process by taking both intrapsychic and interpersonal factors into consideration.

4.4.1 A developmental diagnosis

There is no satisfactory nosological classification of children's emotional disorders. The GAP report on the Diagnostic Process in Child Psychiatry (1957) recommends that "whenever possible a clinical diagnosis should be made," but it also recognizes that "with children in a developmental state, such classification is often difficult since the clinical entities are not clearly defined." [24].

A panel on child analysis (1963), reported by Neubauer [32], had addressed itself to the task of formulating a classification based on developmental principles and recommended four broad categories: (1) development as a measure of health and pathology, (2) developmental disorders, (3) disorders in the continuum between normal conflict and pathology, and (4) primary disturbances and their effect on development. The first one of these categories (development as a measure of health and pathology) was formulated after years of study in the Hampstead Clinic and was the one which, since its initial presentation, had received the greatest attention from child-analysts and child-psychotherapists alike. Its promise for a developmental classification is due primarily to the fact that it is directed toward the assessment of the child's health, as well as toward his pathology. The assessment draws attention to deviations from the norm before these may crystallize into symptoms.

The concept of the "developmental lines" I provide the therapist with points of orientation which can best serve the assessment of the child's total personality. The lines of development, as from "sucking to rational eating" or from "wetting and soiling to bladder control," "are far from being theoretical abstractions … they are rather historical realities, which when assembled, convey a convincing picture of an individual child's personal achievement, or, on the other hand, of his failures in personality development. The developmental lines reflect the result of the interaction between drive and ego-superego development and their reaction to environmental influences, i.e., between maturation, adaptation, and structuralization." [1].

The same developmental principles which Anna Freud employed toward the formulation of the developmental lines, namely, maturation, adaptation, and structuralization, can be used not only in the assessment of the individual child, but also as guidelines toward the formulation of broad clinical categories of childhood disorders. Such categories would have to be broad enough to include the widest possible range of clinical manifestations. Based on developmental principles, the value of these categories would not be on the traditional ordering of the disorders but primarily in relation to the planning of therapeutic action.

Maturation refers to the rate of physical and physiological development which contributes the constitutional factors to emotional development. My discussion will focus on the diagnostic significance of structuralization and adaptation and not touch on the issue of maturation.

Structuralization refers to the development of the psychic agencies with their relatively independent and autonomous functions. Structures have to be differentiated from ad hoc psychic functioning. Ad hoc functioning may take place according to either primary or secondary process. "When a particular form of discharge becomes regular and habitual, a structure has been formed which regulates the discharge of what was at first either primary-or-secondary process ad hoc discharge. Once a structure has been formed, it constitutes a fixed organization, so that neither the structure nor the function it regulates undergoes any change." [25]. In terms of development, this refers to the progressive differentiation of the psyche into the structure of the ego, id, and superego. Clinically, the degree of structuralization is reflected in the relative stability and secondary autonomy which ego and superego functions had achieved. For example, in the immature mind, regression following psychic trauma effects those ego functions which have been acquired last and which therefore had achieved the least stability. Ego regression and the failure of certain ego functions to develop (speech, secondary process thinking, reality testing) indicate serious weakness in the child's psychic organization. Similarly, it is of developmental-diagnostic significance to evaluate the degree of autonomy which the superego, as a relatively independent psychic structure, had achieved.

In many childhood disorders, ego and superego functions had attained considerable structuralization and autonomy, and the child is still not able to utilize these functions adequately. A failure to use adequately developed ego functions is due to insufficient narcissistic cathexis of these functions. The adequate narcissistic cathexis of the ego functions, be they physical or intellectual, promote the child's sense of self-cohesiveness. The close relationship between the experience of a cohesive, unitary self as a consequence of sufficient narcissistic cathexis and a well-functioning ego has been clearly stated by Kohut: "Narcissistic cathexis of the self-image is an important precondition for a cohesively functioning ego; that by contrast, the absence of such a cathexis tends to lead to disordered ego functions." [7]. Similarly, failure in the narcissistic cathexis of the superego leaves the child narcissistically vulnerable to his environment since he remains dependent on them for the regulation of his self-esteem. A developmental diagnosis has to include the assessment of the degree of narcissistic cathexis of the self (and ego and superego functions) as this finds expression in the child's pleasure and enthusiasm for his activities, his self-esteem, and his ability to cope with narcissistic injuries.

The recognition of self-pathology in adults will eventually expand our knowledge related to the clinical manifestations of the failure in the transformation of narcissism in children. The pathology of the self[5] in children results in manifestations similar to those in adults; lack of initiative, zest, or enthusiasm and a lack of guiding ideals for the future. The importance of the self, developmentally and in the formation of psychopathology, has recently been thoroughly discussed from a new vantage point, namely from the reconstruction in adult analysis, by Kohut [7, 8]. In this context, in the grouping of childhood disorders into broad categories, it is helpful to remember that "In the narcissistic personality disorders, we deal not with gross structural defects in a particular ego function or with superego lacunae – though such may occur – but rather with the lack of narcissistic cathexis of these structures. It is the narcissistic cathexis of the ego and superego functions which determines the degree to which these functions are experienced as part of a cohesive self." [26]. While the developmental diagnosis of structural defects (gross and/ or narcissistic) provides us with a metapsychological view of the psychotic, borderline, and narcissistic personality disorders, the mode of adaptation, particularly the degree of internalization which the adaptive mechanisms had undergone, provides us with a view of the neurotic disorders in children. Adaptation, in the context used by Anna Freud, refers to both healthy and pathological forms of adaptations. Since "adaptation" in the literature usually refers only to healthy patterns in the personality, I shall speak of "pathological solutions" when referring to neurotic compromise formations. In making a developmental diagnosis in a child, it is equally important to state the degree to which the adaptive mechanisms or pathological solutions have become internalized, as it is to spell out the specific contents of the defensive and adaptive mechanisms. The degree of internalization of conflicts, defenses, pathological and healthy identifications, determines the degree to which a child is no longer open to the therapeutic or pathological influences of his environment. Since the child's psyche remains an "open system" well into latency and sometimes beyond, it is characteristic of the neurotic disorders of children to be, in a way, "straddling" between solutions which the child had reached intrapsychically and solutions which are tied to parental attitudes and responses. The degree of internalization is closely linked to the degree of structuralization; conflicts and their neurotic solutions can only develop in a psyche which had fairly well differentiated into its separate (ego, id, and superego) structures.

Using these four developmental principles, (A) maturation, (B) the degree of structuralization (C) the narcissistic cathexis of the self, and (D) the degree of internalization of neurotic solutions, we find that the emotional disorders of children fall essentially into three large categories. These categories are best conceptualized on a continuum; at either end of the continuum, we observe the extreme forms of the particular disorder, while in the middle we find the combinations and the variations of the two extremes.

(1) The first extreme form of pathology is exhibited by a group of children who present themselves with syndromes which had resulted from failures in ego differentiation, along with various degrees of constitutional factors. These children suffer from serious developmental ·arrests with various degrees to total interruption of personality development. (Anaclitic depression [27], atypical child [28], autistic-symbiotic psychosis [29], maternal deprivation [30], and childhood schizophrenia [31].)

(2) At the other end of the continuum are children who, after the structuralization of an adequately differentiated ego, developed neurotic solutions which were relatively well-contained within their psychic structures. Though the psyche of these children can no longer be considered an "open system," the internalization of neurotic solutions, as mentioned earlier, is a relative matter in the preadolescent child.

(3) The third and largest group of children, in the middle of the continuum, is of special interest to the therapist since here the diagnosis is not as clear-cut as in either of the two previous groups. In this middle group, we may find any combination of all four of the developmental factors manifested in the same child. (A) Structuralization, which is not absent, but defective; the ego functions have attained relative, age-appropriate autonomy, but are labile and prone to regression. Similarly, the superego functions may be tenuous or defective (superego lacunae). (B) The narcissistic cathexis of the self, while sufficient to prevent permanent fragmentation, is not sufficient to provide the child with a sense of cohesiveness, with optimal functioning, and the enjoyment of his activities. The structural defects due to inadequate narcissistic cathexis of the self may be primarily responsible for the lack· of initiative in these children, as well as for their inability to use their ideals as reliable guides for their actions. (C) The neurotic solutions, though partially internalized, are still predominantly linked to, and are responsive to, the attitudes of the environment. Examples are those children, usually diagnosed as suffering from neurotic behavior disorders, whose neurotic conflicts are not contained by internalized neurotic symptoms, but rather acted out in behavior which involves the child's environment. The environment usually becomes involved by the projection of guilt, by attempts at mutual control, and by covert and overt expressions of hostility.

Using these broad developmental categories, we now have to answer the question, which form of treatment would ideally be responsive to each of these groups of patients? In the first group of children with syndromes resulting from lack of adequate ego differentiation, changed parental attitudes have a limited therapeutic effect. These children are usually placed into a therapeutic milieu away from home, since their serious developmental arrests may not be reversible. They may be helped to achieve no more than some rudimentary form of object relationship. In these cases, the environment carries the total therapeutic responsibility, as treatment aims at structure building in an optimally frustrating environment. It has not yet been conclusively proven whether or not the most carefully designed therapeutic milieu can indeed reverse the more severe forms of these developmental arrests.

The second group of children at the other end of the continuum, with the advanced degree of internalization of pathological solutions to their conflicts, are also limited in their ability to respond to a therapeutic milieu within the home but for a different reason. These children do not respond to the therapeutic attitude of their home environment because they live in a transference relationship with their own parents. This means that the child continues to perceive and to respond to the parent of his earlier (traumatic) childhood. These children are ideally treated by methods which permit the development of transferences, that is; either in psychoanalysis or in intensive psychotherapy. The parents, under these circumstances, may or may not participate in the treatment process. However, as I mentioned earlier, even under these circumstances, the home must provide a therapeutic milieu so as not to interfere with the child's progress in treatment.

What are our technical options for the third group of children, the ones in the middle of the continuum; children who suffer from various degrees of structural defects (either narcissistic or object libidinal) and from partially internalized solutions to their-neurotic conflicts? Since in this group, the child's psychopathology is closely linked to his environment, both in terms of the nature of the conflict and in terms of the structural defect, treatment without a therapeutic milieu in the home is not likely to succeed. The manner in which such a milieu is created has been described in the previous sections.

If parental pathology does not interfere with their ability to respond empathically to the therapist's translation of the meaning of the child's behavior, periodic consultation with or without the child's presence is usually sufficient. However, if parental pathology interlocks with the child's pathology, the parents may need individual help in order to help them develop an empathic, therapeutic attitude toward the child. As far as the child is concerned, the more firmly internalization of pathological solutions has been established, the more likely the need for individual treatment. Structural defects, on the other hand, require the participation of the environment to a greater degree. In addition to the considerations which are based on the nature and extent of the parents' pathology, variations as to who will be in what form of treatment is determined by the motivation of the individual members of the family. It is not the person who is in greatest need of treatment who will necessarily carry the greatest burden of therapy. Frequently, compromise solutions have to be found when either child or one of the parents refuses to participate in the treatment process.

4.4.2 The concept of the single process and the use of a model

The processing of psychological data is a challenging task under all circumstances, but this is particularly true when the therapist has to integrate clinical material generated by more than one person. In the treatment of children, the processing of data and the overall therapeutic task can be greatly facilitated when the different aspects of the treatment are conceptualized as a single process. This is possible if the material the participants produce (one or both parents, with or without the participation of the child) is consistently related and interpreted to the child's psychopathology.

In individual therapy, the process of treatment is characterized by the sequential unfolding of certain experiences within the doctor-patient relationship. These are experiences which are phase-specific for the process – the initial phase being characterized by mutual assessment between therapist and patient, the middle phase by the crystallization of the conflicts and defenses and their working through, and the termination by the resolution of the unique relationship between therapist and patient.

The same sequence should be recognizable when more than one person makes a contribution to the evolution of the process. Conceptualizing the treatment of a child and his emotional environment as evolving within a single process is supported by the observation that various aspects of the treatment are usually contributed by the various members of the family: (A) while it is the child's symptom, it is the parents' motivation for change which brings the family for professional help; (B). the therapeutic alliance is based on initial parental motivation which eventually has to evolve to include all participants in the treatment process (In cases where the parents are not motivated and they are reluctantly complying with an outside referral, no meaningful therapeutic process will be set into motion. The therapeutic task then has to focus on the question of motivation.); (C) while the child's capacity to utilize insight is limited, the parents, in order to effect changes in themselves in relation to the child, have to achieve considerable insight into their own and into the nature of the child's difficulties.

Conceptualizing the treatment of the parents and the symptomatic child as occurring in a single process will not permit the therapist an artificial separation into "diagnosis" and "treatment." The therapist cannot loose sight of what the parents' needs are therapeutically while he is asking their help in diagnosing the child. Diagnosis and treatment may be conceptually differentiated in the therapist's mind. For any patient, treatment begins when he first makes up his mind to seek professional help. From the beginning, the therapist has to be mindful of the patient's position in the total process, whether the child or any member of his family is the patient.

Assembling a developmental history in the first interview may distract the therapist from his primary task of engaging the parents into the treatment process. This is most effectively achieved by exploring the parents own understanding regarding the child's problems and the efforts they had made so far to resolve them. In the later phases of the treatment, with the focus on the child, the therapist will tune in on and respond interpretively to those aspects in the parents' personality which unconsciously interlock, and therefore support, the child's pathology.

The use of a model could further facilitate the processing of the data and its conceptualization as a single process. Models, fashioned according to the various concepts related to the workings of the mind, have been extremely useful in facilitating the processing of psychoanalytic data. Theoretical concepts such as the structural theory have been made easier to grasp by the use of the tripartite model. Similarly, the topographic model has illuminated the theory of the mind in its stratification into the conscious, preconscious, and unconscious systems. There have been several attempts at the pictoral representation of the self–object theory as well. Models are the graphical representation of ideas, a picture of what would otherwise have to be a lengthy description of a complex theory. As theories change in order to accommodate new knowledge, new models are added as tools of conceptualization.

I am proposing a model which would facilitate the conceptualization of the treatment process and its relationship to the nature of the child's psychopathology. This model would serve the following purposes. (1) It would help the therapist to separate formulations which are based on the intrapsychic experiences of the parents and the child from those which are based on interpersonal behavior and modes of communication. The model would have to indicate the intricate relationship between intrapsychic experiences and their interpersonal ramifications. (Throughout this paper, I have referred to the child's "emotional environment;" this not only includes the parents, the siblings, and important members of the extended family to the child, as well as the child's teachers, but it also includes the nature of the parental relationship. This is indicated on the model by an arrow between the parents). (2) The relative "openness" of the child's psyche would have to be indicated in the model, since special emphasis is placed on the influence of parental attitudes on the child, both developmentally and therapeutically. At the same time, the presence of the child's ongoing, though limited, effect on the parent(s) has to be indicated on the model as well. (3) The model also would have to express the aims of the treatment which is to resolve the interpersonal conflicts and thereby help establish empathic communication between parent and child. Such a model is presented in Figure 4.1.

The entanglement of the threads represents the interpersonal conflicts created by the interaction between parents and child. Though the parents may not react to the child in unison, and siblings and other members of the environment may participate in the interpersonal conflict, the single knot located between parent and child indicates the overwhelming importance which this particular interaction has on the child's psychopathology and his emotional development. For example, if a child has to make intrapsychic compromises to deal with strong rivalrous affects related to one of his siblings, this would be indicated with a dot inside the circle which outlines the child's psyche. The emotional environment in which sibling rivalry will either dissipate in the course of development or become the source of internal compromise formations, depends primarily on parental attitudes toward the child.

The knot is created by threads, the roots of which belong to the psyche of the child and to the psyche of the parents. In normal development, the threads, which are the lines of conscious and unconscious attitudes and communication patterns, run uninterruptedly between parent and child. The knot is created· by the neurotic entanglement of the threads, thereby interfering with the normal parental function of supporting and facilitating the child's emotional growth.

In processing clinical data, the image of a single knot helps the therapist(s) to select out those features in the child's emotional environment which are most crucially related to his psychopathology and, therefore, most importantly interfere with his progressive development. The intrapsychic pathology of the parents, if not directly related to the child's, does not make a contribution to the interpersonal threads which create the knot. The focus on the child's psychopathology calls for a selective approach to the parents' emotional life.

In terms of the representation of the child's psyche, I want to indicate two essential points: (A) the degree of structuralization and differentiation and (B) the degree of internalization of pathological compromise formations and identifications. The degree of structuralization and differentiation is represented in the broken line delineating the child's psyche from the environment. This suggests the extent to which the child's psyche is still open. Internalizations are either complete (inside the child's psyche) or incomplete (on the periphery of the child's psyche). The child's psychopathology is expressed by

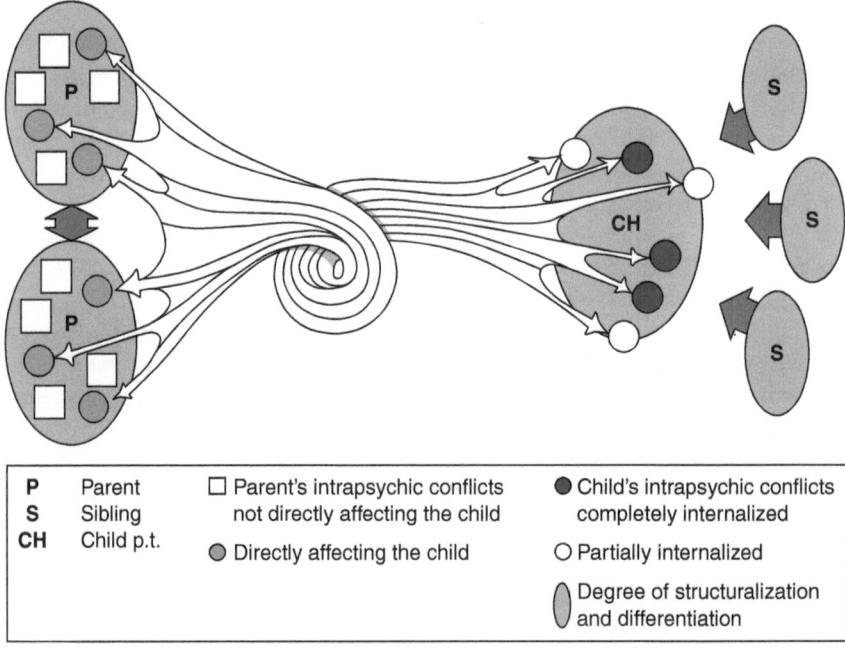

P Parent	☐ Parent's intrapsychic conflicts not directly affecting the child
S Sibling	
CH Child p.t.	◉ Directly affecting the child

● Child's intrapsychic conflicts completely internalized

○ Partially internalized

◖ Degree of structuralization and differentiation

Figure 4.1 Model of conceptualization [32, 33].

the combination of the degree of structuralization with that of partial or total internalization of pathological conflict solutions and identifications.

The therapeutic aim is to untangle the knot so that the lines of interpersonal communications can again run smoothly. The smooth running of the threads facilitates the resolution of the child's conflicts which had become completely or partially internalized. Untangling the knot does not mean that the threads which created it will be disconnected. The opposite is true; only a sense of secure connectedness with his emotional environment permits a child to resolve his conflicts and to continue his developmental progress. The child's developmental progress eventually results in the gradual disengagement of his inner life from that of his emotional milieu. To attempt an emotional separation, either by physical separation or by suggestive means, is to fail to take into consideration that separation can only grow out of the safety of a well-established and reliable sense of connectedness with one's emotional environment. This is so, because long after the achievement of cognitive distinction between self and non-self, the child continues to utilize his environment to complete the development of his inner world. Final separation from one's emotional environment does not occur until adolescence or later in life.

Notes

1 The nontherapeutic responses by hospital personnel are frequently referred to as countertransference reactions. However, since these reactions are rarely reactions to the patients transferences but rather direct responses to the patients actual behavior, it is theoretically incorrect to refer to them as countertransferences.
2 In this connection, the question could be raised whether Freud would have been as successful in his treatment of "Little Hans" [10] as he was, had he directly given his interpretations to the child rather than through the child's father. Was it therapeutically·significant that the father understood (with the help of Freud's interpretations) the origin of Little Hans's fear of horses and had thereby empathically accepted the child's Oedipal rage? help of Freud's interpretations) the origin of Little Hans's fear of horses and had·thereby empathically accepted the child's Oedipal rage?
3 "The therapeutic process refers to the intrapsychic and interpersonal experiences of the patient, mobilized in the therapist-patient relationship, in response to the patient's inner needs and the therapist's interventions. The therapeutic·process encompasses both the nonspecific (empathy, nonjudgmental attitude) and the specific (conflict resolution, transmuting internalization) curative factors." [15].
4 I am grateful to Ms. Merrilee Atkins for permitting me to use this case vignette.
5 "The self, as a comparative experience – near psychoanalytic abstraction, is central to all human experience since it contains man's nuclear ambitions and ideals which are amalgamated to the sense of continuity and cohesion of (our) body and mind" (Kohut, unpublished manuscript, 1975).

References

1 Freud A: Normality and Pathology in Childhood. New York, International Universities Press, 1965, p. 64
2 Weiss S: Parameters in child analysis. J Am Psychoanal Assoc 12:587–599, 1964

3 Carek D: Principles or Child Psychotherapy. Springfield, III. Charles C Thomas, 1972, p. 25

4 Winnicott D W: Therapeutic Consultations in Children Psychiatry. New York, Basic Books, 1971, p. 5

5 Gottschalk LA, Brown SB, Bruney EH, et al: An evaluation of a parent's group in childcentered clinic. Psychiatry 36:157–171, 1973

6 Kohut H: Introspection, empathy, and psychoanalysis. J AM Psychoanal Assoc 7:459–483, 1959

7 Kohut H: The Analysis of the Self. New York, International Universities Press, 1971, p. 132

8 Kohut H: The psychoanalyst in the community of scholars. Address given at the University of Cincinnati, November 15, 1973 (in press)

9 Olden, C.: On adult empathy with children. Psychoanal Study Child 8:111–125, 1953

10 Freud, S.: Analysis of a phobia in a five-year-old-boy in: Standard Edition, vol X. 1909, pp. 5–149

11 Krug O, Stuart BL: Collaborative treatment of mother and boy with fecal retention, soiling, and a school phobia, in Gardner GE (ed.): Case Studies in Childhood Emotional Disabilities, vol II, 1954, pp. 1–28

12 Hallowitz. D: A collaborative diagnostic and treatment process with parents. Social Case-work 3:76–96, 1958

13 Hartman N, Horn P: Collaborative treatment as a therapeutic tool. Social Case-work 39:459–463, 1958

14 Szurek S: Some problems in collaborative therapy. Newsletter Am Assoc Psych Soc Work 9:1–7, 1940

15 Ornstein P, Ornstein A: On the continuing evolution of psychoanalytic psychotherapy: Reflections upon recent trends and some predictions for the future. The Tenth Annual Symposium on Psychotherapy, Boston, Mass., April 1975 (unpublished manuscript)

16 Whitaker C: A family therapist looks at marital therapy, in Gurman AS, Rice DG (eds): Couples in Conflict. 1975, p. 169, 166

17 Bell JE: Family Therapy. New York, Aronson, 1975, p. 17, 18

18 Bowen M: Toward the differentiation of self in one's family of origin, in Andres F, Lorio J (eds): Georgetown Family Symposia, vol 1, 1971–1972, p. 86

19 Bloch D, La Perriere K: Techniques of family therapy: A conceptual frame, in Bloch D (ed.): Techniques of Family Psychotherapy. New York, Grune & Stratton, 1973, pp. 1–19

20 Minuchin S: Conflict resolution family therapy. Psychiatry 28:278–286, 1965

21 Jackson D: The question of family homeostasis. Psychiatr Q 31:79–90, 1957

22 Satir V: Conjoint Family Therapy, Palo Alto, Science and Behavior Books, 1964

23 Ackerman N, Papp P, Prosky P: Childhood disorders and interlocking pathology in family relationships, in Anthony EJ, Kouperni KC (eds): The Child and His Family. New York, Wiley-Interscience, 1970, pp. 241–265

24 Group for the Advancement of Psychiatry (GAP): The Diagnostic Process in Child Psychiatry. Reprint 38, 1957, p. 343

25 Gill M: Topography and systems in psychoanalytic theory. Psychol Issues Monograph 10. New York, International Universities Press, 1963, p. 113

26 Ornstein A: The dread to repeat and the new beginning: A contribution to the psychoanalysis of the narcissistic personality disorders, in: The Annual of Psychoanalysis, vol II. New York, International Universities Press, 1974, p. 238

27 Spitz R: Anaclitic depression: An inquiry into the genesis of psychiatric conditions in early childhood. Psychoanal Study Child 2:315–342, 1946

28 Rank B: A clinical contribution to early ego development. Psychoanal Study Child 5:53–65, 1950

29 Mahler M: On symbiotic child psychosis: Genetic, dynamic and restitutive. Psychoanal Study Child 10:195–212, 1955

30 Bowlby J: Grief and mourning in infancy and early childhood. Psychoanal Study Child 15:9–52, 1960

31 Goldfarb W: Childhood Schizophrenia. Cambridge, Harvard University Press, 1961

32 Neubauer P: Psychoanalytic contributions to the nosology of childhood psychic disorders. J Am Psychoanal Assoc 11:595–604, 1963

33 Ornstein A, Ornstein P: On the interpretive process in psychoanalysis. Int J Psychoanal Psychother 4:219–271, 1975

5 Parenting as a function of the adult self

A psychoanalytic developmental perspective

Anna Ornstein and Paul Ornstein

Once human behavior became the legitimate subject of scientific inquiry around the turn of the twentieth century, infant and child development studies had become central to these research endeavors. Today, there is a great deal of literature related to the study of infants, young children, and the early phases of mothering. Indeed, the most revealing and dependable data on mothering currently available are from the burgeoning literature on infant research. The findings on parenting in these mother-infant studies, although secondary to the data from the infant studies, are of great significance because they fairly consistently support an evolutionary biological disposition for mothering. In the early phases of mothering, a biological readiness appears to complement the infant's "built-in" capacity to solicit social responses from the environment. "The mother is involved in a natural process with her baby, a process that unfolds with a fascinating intricacy and complexity for which she and her baby are well prepared by the millennia of evolution" [46].

The most persistent supporters of a biological readiness for mothering have been Klaus and Kennell [26], Ainsworth [2], and Bowlby [13]. They maintained that only civilization and technology obscure the mother's instincts that could otherwise guide her in successful bonding and attachment to her infant. As with other mammals, these authors believe bonding and attachment have to occur at certain "critical periods" in the infant's life and that in the human these experiences have far-reaching consequences for later development, specifically for that of language and intelligence. However, this biological readiness, the capacity for bonding and attachment, remain disputed motives for parenting even during infancy and certainly beyond the earliest phases of the infant's life [15, 17, 41].

Benedek, whose studies of the development of motherliness are the most widely accepted by psychoanalysts, found that in the human female mothering behavior has two sources: one is rooted in her physiology; "the other evolved as an expression of her personality which had developed under environmental influences that could modify her motherliness" [10].

Although we agree with Benedek in the essential aspects of her observation, we wish to add that the biological roots of motherliness of the human female may not only be "modified," but may actually be outweighed or totally overshadowed by psychological factors. And while the biological and physiological factors may still be in evidence in relationship to the infant, it will be the mother's psychology, "the expression of her personality which has developed under environmental influences," that will determine her responsiveness to the increasingly more complex developmental needs of her child.

In our modern Western society, the mother (if she is to care for the child at all) may be only one member of a group of adults engaged in the care of a particular child. From the child's perspective, it may be more appropriate to speak of a "parenting unit" defined as one person (e.g., either parent) or a group of persons from whom the child can receive or extract the responses he needs for his development; to be a "mother" or a "father" is not synonymous with parenting. By introducing the notion of a "parenting unit," we do not intend to minimize the importance that the primary caretaker has in a fundamental achievement of the psyche, namely, attachment. Attachment and bonding appear to occur within the first ten days of the infant's life; within the first week, the newborn shows preference for the mother's smell, voice, and familiar appearance [33]. However, we wish to draw attention to the infant's (and child's) capacity to elicit social responsiveness from a variety of people and pets in the environment and thereby imperceptibly compensate for the unavailable primary caretaker. In this chapter, our attention is not on the disturbance in the capacity for attachment in the "primary caretaker" but on parenting in general-parenting that is not restricted to the early years of the child's life but encompasses the entire parental life cycle.

We find the concept of a parenting unit particularly useful in assessing the development of children who grow up in multiple foster homes, in divorced or "reconstituted" families, or under other unconventional circumstances. Clinicians cannot readily find an explanation for the capacity of these children not only to cope with some very obvious life stresses, but for them to continue their progressive development. Rather than attributing such resiliency to unidentified constitutional factors, although these may perhaps play apart, we are suggesting that children are able to extract developmentally needed "selfobject responses"[1] from an environment that, to an external observer, may appear to have no redeeming features. And the obverse may be true as well: an environment that, to an external observer, may be "average expectable," may nevertheless not be responsive to a particular child's developmental needs. It is, therefore, understandable that no direct correlation can be made between a particular emotional illness of the parent and that parent's parental capacities or dysfunctions; however, some parental disturbances are more likely to create overt symptoms in the child, while others are more likely to create covert symptoms. Still others, under similar circumstances, may "develop a brittle normality or even super-normality" [3].

Because predictions for psychological development cannot be made by the "objective" assessment of the child's environment, it is important to make a distinction between an *etiological* and a *genetic* approach to the investigations of parenting. Data obtained from the direct investigation of parents in the course of psychoanalysis and psychotherapy have etiological significance for child development and psychopathology, while data regarding parenting that is obtained from the treatment of the child (or adult) are of genetic significance. Kohut [27] differentiated the etiological from the genetic approach: "The genetic approach in psychoanalysis relates to the investigation of those subjective psychological experiences of the child which usher in a chronic change in the distribution and further development of the endopsychic forces and structures. The etiological approach, on the other hand, relates to the investigation of those objectively ascertainable factors which, in interaction with the child's psyche as it is constituted at a given moment, may or may not elicit the genetically decisive experiences."

In our conceptualization of parenting, we have used both sources of information. The treatment of children and the psychoanalysis of adults have provided insight into parenting that was derived from reconstructions (the genetic approach). This has elucidated the subjective experiences of the children in relation to their parents. On the other hand, the simultaneous treatment of parents and children has provided us with a view of the "objectively ascertainable factors" of interaction (the etiological approach). It is in this latter context that we can appreciate the ongoing mutuality and reciprocity that exists between the child and his emotional environment. We have found Kohut's theory of the self and the development of the self within an empathically responsive selfobject environment to be the most useful tool for the ordering of our data in all of these treatment modalities.

5.1 Adaptation, development, and pathogenesis

We are putting forward the view that parenting can only be assessed in conjunction with the assessment of a particular child, since focusing on the parent alone provides the clinician only with an etiological perspective. It is only through the immersion into the child's inner world that the clinician can also appreciate what has become genetically significant for a particular child from the many, possibly significant parental influences. Parenting is a dynamic activity; its mutuality and reciprocity with the child's inner world has thus far been encompassed by the concept of adaptation, which was articulated by Hartmann [24].

Hartmann's seminal work on "Ego Psychology and the Problem of Adaptation" [24] favored the concept of reciprocity in the process of adaptation. In psychoanalysis today, this concept has been replaced by one that considers the individual's response to the environment as either alloplastic or autoplastic. This either/or view of adaptation has been perpetuated because of the relatively rigid conceptual separation of the psychoneuroses (the result of autoplastic adaptation) from the "acting out" forms of psychopathology that have been viewed as aiming at an alloplastic adaptation. Hartmann's statement that "adaptation is primarily a reciprocal relationship between the organism and its environment" [24] has not remained in central focus in the subsequent psychoanalytic literature and neither has the statement he made regarding "the average not expectable environment": "The degree of adaptiveness can only be determined with reference to environmental situations (average expectable – i.e., typical – situations, or on the average not expectable – i.e., atypical – situations)."

It is our view that the notion of a not expectable (i.e., atypical) situation has not found its way into psychoanalytic thinking. By maintaining, at least for theoretical purposes, that the external environment is "average expectable" (i.e., invariant), analysts can focus more exclusively on what they consider to be only internal variations. This focus has undoubtedly permitted a more thorough appreciation of the internally generated, drive-related conflicts and their underlying unconscious fantasies as motives for normal development and as sources of anxiety and symptom formation. However, this sharp dichotomy between external and internal can only be maintained by the unwarranted assumption of the presence of a consensually valid external reality (at least operationally). Hartmann [24], discussing the interplay between psychological and biological factors in development, asked: "Are the exogenous factors the average expectable kind (family situation, mother-child relationship and others), or are the environmental conditions of a different sort? In other words, the question is whether, and to what extent, a certain course of development can count on average expectable stimulations (environmental releasers) and whether, and to what extent, and in what direction it will be deflected by environmental influences of a different sort."

Anthony [4] discussed the historical antecedents of the psychoanalyst's ambivalence toward the external environment, specifically the resistance to considering the importance of the family in the child's analysis. He says that to consider the family in a child's analysis "is tantamount to becoming an environmentalist, the modern equivalent of the 'wild analyst.'" In order to facilitate the psychoanalyst's treatment of the child and still take into account the child's complex experiences of his or her emotional environment, Anthony suggested that the analyst should recognize that the child constructs three forms of "families" in his psyche, to which gets added a fourth one – the one the child constructs in the course of analysis. "The various families – the intrapsychic oedipal one, the idealized representational one, the actual interpersonal one, and the analyst's hypothetical one – may all appear in symbolic play with the family figures provided by the analyst." The analyst's task is to disentangle these various "families" and to appraise the family realistically; at the same time, he or she should encourage the formation of the imaginary family via the transference.

In other words, the child analyst, by assessing the family's "reality," has to disentangle the intricate impact of the family on the child's psyche and the child's own contribution to the pathological interactions. Once this has been accomplished, the analyst is expected to help the child separate the family's real impact from his or her own oedipal wishes and fantasies. The reality of the family and its impact on the child is conceived here as something that has become "superimposed" on the unconscious oedipal fantasies, which, once exposed, becomes the legitimate subject of the analyst's interpretations.

Although this recommendation is broadly encompassing, two questions must be raised: Is the analyst in the position to appraise "the reality" of the family and is the child able to separate experientially "the interpersonal family from her internalized libidinal and ego attitudes?" [4].

The question as to what external or internal factors account for pathogenicity has been with psychoanalysts ever since Freud's time. Freud's original answer to this dilemma was the introduction of the concept of the "complemental series" [22]. This concept was to explain the pathogenesis of the adult forms of psychoneuroses; it meant that traumatic events in a child's life created libidinal fixations, which, when reactivated later in life, lead to neurotic compromise formations. Such neurotic compromises require the presence of a well-developed ego and superego. For this reason, neurotic conditions, based on the vicissitudes of the Oedipus complex, had been traditionally differentiated from "deficiency illnesses." The deficiency in the child's ego and superego structure has been related either to gross parental neglect, physical abuse, institutionalization, or other, as yet unknown, factors that have prevented children from using the environment effectively, thus possibly leading to childhood psychosis.

In clinical practice, child therapists have long recognized another group of patients – children who do not suffer from the consequences of an unresolved Oedipus complex and who do not exhibit gross structural defects because of severe parental neglect or abuse. These are children who suffer from the consequences of various degrees of discreet structural deficits that can be related to equally discreet and subtle failures in parental empathy. Kohut's discovery of the selfobject transferences has alerted child therapists to those parental functions that, because of their silent presence, by and large have been taken for granted. We are referring to the infant's and child's ongoing developmental need for validation and the need to merge first with the parents' physical strength and power and later with their moral strength and power. These parental functions do not simply "facilitate" a "drive-determined" sequence in development, but rather, they themselves are responsible for the building up of psychic structures by becoming transmutedly internalized [27, 47].

Infant research had repeatedly demonstrated that the capacity to elicit life-sustaining environmental responses that are crucial for the infant's momentary functioning and for the building up of permanent psychic structures are inborn. The infant, born with "a predictable genetic ground plan" [32], has to be assured of phase-appropriate environmental responses. These are the responses that self psychology calls "selfobject functions." Sander [43], for example, spoke of a "fitting together" of the endogenous (infant-determined) and exogenous (caretaker-determined) influences. The fitting together is a developmental accomplishment that requires the caretaker's ability "to read" the infant's clues. The process of fitting together that Sander also conceptualized as an "interactional schema" (similar to Piaget's sensorimotor schemata) has a high level of reciprocity in the process of adaptation.

Sander [43] used the model of adaptation to account for the two major aspects of personality development: integration and differentiation. These two, seemingly opposing directions in the development of the individual, occur within the same contextual unit and, therefore, they have to be accounted for by the same theoretical model. For example, the increasing differentiation of the child's emotional, cognitive, and perceptual capacities have to become integrated into the very same system in which this differentiation has taken place in order for these capacities to achieve functional freedom. In other words, functional freedom is not achieved by the child extricating himself from "the interactive regulative system" in which he is embedded and of which he is a part, but by achieving new levels of adaptation with increasing complexity within that very same system. The sequence in this interactive regulatory system is described by Sander [43].

With one component, the infant, rapidly growing and consequently rapidly changing, new qualities and quantities of infant behavior are constantly being introduced into the content of interaction. The regulation of infant functions, based on behaviors that have become harmoniously coordinated between mother and infant, will become perturbed with the advent of each new, and usually more specifically focused and intentionally initiated activity of the growing infant. Thus adaptation or mutual modification on a new level is required. Since the behavioral innovations by the infant are often aimed at a progressive assumption of control of situations as a part of the widening of his scope of self-regulation vis-á-vis the environment (i.e., he becomes more vigorously alloplastic), these changes impinge critically on the mother's long-established strategies of self-regulation (p. 135).

Our focus is on the parents' capacity to respond to the challenge of this impingement on their "long-established strategies of self-regulation" in relationship to the rapidly growing and, therefore, rapidly changing psychological organization of the child. This focus on parental responsiveness, however, ought not be interpreted as placing the sole responsibility of a child's development on the caretaker's capacity to pick up the growing child's clues for what should be a perfectly empathic response. We agree with Greenspan [23] that each organism has its "individual way of processing, organizing and differentiating experiences ... and that the final common pathway is unique to each individual ... suggesting something fundamental about the organism's manner of organizing its experience of its world, internal and external, animate and inanimate."

However, while we agree that each organism has its "individual way of processing, organizing, and differentiating experiences," we question the separation of internal from external experiences as they become integrated into a final common pathway. Rather, we suggest (in keeping with Sander's interaction schemas) that the environment's responses to the child "create" experiences that are unique not only to that child but also to that environment. The experiences that become transmutedly internalized and will constitute the relatively independent tension, affect, and self-esteem regulating systems of the self are being "created" between the infant and his emotional environment in an ongoing way.

The significance of social interaction between infant and caretaker is strongly emphasized by Stern [46]. In presenting a research tool that would measure social interactive behavior and styles, he had commented that such an instrument would have to be used in three ways [6].

> The first is to identify something distinctive about particular parents and see how that factor affects their social interaction with their infants. For example, one could compare mothers who differ along an important clinical parameter such as mental illness. The second use, similarly, is to identify and compare infants as known risks for some developmental deviance. A third use is to explore the nature and ontogeny of the specific fit of particular parents and babies across time to see how they navigate the hurdles of various developmental milestones together.

Infant researchers we have cited so far and others whose work is relevant but too numerous to be quoted bring the primacy of the drives as motivators of development and as providers of psychic energy into serious question; the biological equipment for human psychological development appears to reside in the infant's capacity to elicit certain responses from the environment crucial for his development (i.e., the "selfobject functions" of self psychology). In addition, these researchers in their careful attention to the infant's and child's emotional environment have expanded our view of development from one in which we could simply trace the acquisition of psychic functions to one in which we can also trace the source of the qualities of these functions (i.e., whether or not the acquired functions are executed with joy or only mechanically). According to Greenspan [23]: "Most importantly, under optimal circumstances we note that the toddler is capable of pleasure in a joyful manner, assertiveness and expressions of protest and anger, all tied together in complex behavioral patterns." Even though Greenspan's observations are guided by classical psychoanalytic theory, we do not believe that affects, such as self-assertiveness, anger, and joy are viewed here as drive derivatives that will have to be further modified and neutralized. Rather, these affects are seen as indicative of increased structuralization of the psyche – a developmental accomplishment that is the result of increasing differentiation of the child's affects within the selfobject matrix [7].

Greenspan's structuralist approach to the study of development is particularly useful for psychoanalysts who consider psychoanalysis as a structural psychology par excellence as did Kohut[2] Greenspan's findings confirm Kohut's assumptions that a failure by the environment to respond to the infant's cues leaves defects behind in the psyche that get "filled in" with defensive and negativistic behavior in order for the infant to remain in contact with his or her life-sustaining environment.

If emerging capacities for contingent interactions in sensorimotor and affective areas are not systematically responded to, developmental progress in the most vulnerable areas may slow down or cease, simply because there is no opportunity for repetitive action sequences or practice (i.e., there is lack of repetitive minimal stimulus nutriment necessary to consolidate these capacities) and we may observe cognitive and interpersonal delays. Secondary apathy, withdrawal, disorganization and/or other regression may follow. Also, an infant who gets no response or an inappropriate response (e.g., he is misread) to his "reaching out" cues may mobilize negativistic responses to achieve a reaction from the environment.

(p. 730)

The process of "fitting together" [43], the need to maintain emotional connection between parent and child at all cost [23], and "exploring the nature and ontogeny of the specific fit of particular parents and babies across time to see how they navigate the hurdles of various developmental milestones together" [6] are not only useful conceptualizations of the complex processes of development but are fundamental to the clinician who has to understand the child's "fit," or adaptation or maladaptation, to a particular emotional environment.

5.2 The concept of the self, the self–selfobject unit, and parental selfobject functions

Kohut's developmental theory of the self is based on his description of the various forms of selfobject transferences: the mirror transference, the alter-ego or twinship transference, and the idealizing transference [27, 28]. In self psychology, just as in classical psychoanalytic theory, hypotheses regarding development are based on the transferences that have been observed in the psychoanalytic situation. This makes the developmental theory of the self a psychoanalytic developmental theory, and its validity, therefore, has to be established at first in the psychoanalytic situation itself. However, scientific rigor requires that validation also occur from outside the situation in which the data have originally been gathered. In psychoanalytic developmental theory, this has traditionally been done by direct observation of infants and young children and by the observation of children and their families in the offices of child analysts and child therapists. The review of current literature regarding infant research indicates a high correlation between Kohut's hypothesis regarding the structure-building function of the empathically responsive (selfobject) environment and the findings of present-day infant researchers.

Child psychotherapists have found with increasing frequency that they treat children who live under varied external circumstances, that is, in average, not expectable, environments. Under these circumstances, child therapists are confronted repeatedly with the question as to how to set up a treatment plan that will optimally address those aspects of the emotional milieu that most crucially impinge on the child's development and on the already existing symptoms. It is no longer sufficient to ask the question whether the weight of the pathology resides primarily within the child or within the environment. Rather, we now need a conceptual tool that addresses the question of the fit between the child and his or her emotional environment. We are suggesting that this conceptual tool is provided by the model of the *self-selfobject* unit.

Using the model of the self-selfobject unit, the clinician can conceptualize the various degrees of failures in parenting beyond the early years of the child's life since empathic selfobject responsiveness remains an essential aspect of development throughout childhood. Using this model in the clinical situation, we can either focus on the child's developing self and assess the manner in which the environment is meeting the child's selfobject needs, or we can reverse the model and determine to what extent and in what manner the parents are using the child to meet their own selfobject needs. The latter use of the model is particularly useful in determining parental self-pathology, which is the most frequent source of failures in parental empathy.

The model of the self-selfobject unit has several advantages for the organization of clinical data. It underlines the importance of having to take into consideration the infinite variations of the environment when making an in-depth psychological assessment of a child's development and/or psychopathology. That is, we now recognize that we cannot assess the state of the child's self without considering the way in which the growing self is experiencing and internalizing its emotional environment. Self and environment constitute an experiential unit; the self cannot be conceptualized without the selfobject environment, nor can the functions of the selfobjects be assessed without taking the effect that these functions have on the self into consideration.

The model of the self-selfobject as an experiential unit highlights why the process of adaptation no longer adequately characterizes human psychological development. Although the concept includes the recognition that it is not only the child's psyche that is changing, but (as a result of a high level of reciprocity) the emotional environment changes in relationship to the growing child as well; the concept of adaptation conveys the idea of two entities adjusting to each other's needs. Even when we conceive of this adjustment not only in terms of externally observable behavioral manifestations, but also in terms of the internally achieved changes, the idea of adaptation still remains the external observer's point of view of what happens between the two independent entities that are being observed. In this context the "average expectable" as well as the "average not expectable" environments are also constructed from the vantage point of the external observer. In contrast, the empathic observer attempts to see and grasp the infant's or child's experiencing of the mother or any parenting figure (i.e., the mirroring or idealized selfobject) and proceeds to describe the events between them in terms of the self-experience of each in relation to the other. A similar idea was expressed by Atwood and Stolorow [5]. "We are contending that every phase in a child's development is best conceptualized in terms of the unique, continuously changing psychological field constituted by the intersection of the child's evolving subjective universe with those of the caretakers.... When the psychological organization of the parent cannot sufficiently accommodate to the changing, phase specific needs of the developing child, then the more malleable and vulnerable psychological structure of the child will accommodate to what is available" (p. 69, italics in the original).

The empathic focus on the experiencing self of the infant or child, and thus on the presence or absence of those phase-appropriate selfobject functions that it needs for its wholesome development, permits us to learn about the genetic impact of parenting on children with a variety of constitutions and special endowments. Conversely, a similar focus on the parent's experiencing of the infant or child permits us to learn about the impact that the rearing of a particular child has on the parent's adult self and on parenting capacities.

By focusing our attention on the experiencing self, the concept of the selfobject directs us to an empathic (i.e., vicariously introspective) mode of observation through which we recognize the particular roles and functions of the other for the attainment and maintenance of the cohesiveness of the self and for its vigor and vitality.[3]

Adaptation becomes a necessity on the part of the infant or growing child when the selfobject functions are unavailable or are faulty. It also is necessary when, instead of the parents being responsive to the selfobject needs of the infant or child, the infant or child needs to be responsive to the parents' own imperative needs for self-affirmation.

The model of the self-selfobject unit also helps us conceptualize the various degrees of parental dysfunctions that are related to the parent's own self-development. By focusing on the parent's self, the clinician can determine in what manner and to what extent the parent is using the child as a selfobject in order to maintain his or her fragile self and/or bolster shaky self-esteem.

The usefulness of the model is related to the fact that in the parentchild relationship, both parties, parent and child, fulfill selfobject functions for each other. While the central importance of parental selfobject functions for the child's development can readily be appreciated, the selfobject functions that children serve for the enhancement of the parent's adult self are more difficult to conceptualize. The difficulty lies in the fact that a parent's "average expectable" narcissistic investment in a child may not be readily distinguishable from the subtle ways in which a child may be used for the maintenance of the parent's self-cohesion, or more frequently, for the regulation of self-esteem.

The conception and birth of a child "reopen" adult self-development and constitute a potential for further consolidation and expansion of the adult self. This further expansion is possible because the narcissistic (selfobject) elements are inherent in the parent-child tie. The same idea was originally expressed by Benedek [12] and restated by Lax [30]. "During pregnancy a marked shift toward libidinal concentration on the self occurs. This narcissism, which cathects the expanding self-representation, enables the pregnant woman to feel that the growing body within her constitutes an integral part of herself. In addition to this physical sense of being merged, the pregnant woman day-dreams about her future child and in her fantasy molds it according to her wishes and ego-ideals."

From the time of conception, parental hopes and expectations are experi-enced and later unconsciously conveyed to the child, which not only shape the child's self, but simultaneously firm up the parents' sense of continuity across the generations. Erikson [19] spoke of a "procreative drive" that is part of adult generativity: "... generativity which is concerned with new beings as well as new products and new ideas and which, as a link between the genera-tions, *is as indispensable for the renewal of the adult generation's own life as it is for that of the next generation.*"

If parental hopes and expectations are not conveyed with regard to the child's innate skills and talents, they do not have structure-building properties. For example, praise and enthusiasm in response to a particular behavior that is not experienced by the child as an expression of his or her nuclear self are not empathic responses; such responses are more likely expressions of the parents' own expectations than an affirmation and validation of the child's own self.

Kohut's conceptualization of the selfobject functions may be compared to Winnicott's description of the "facilitating environment" and the concept of the "good-enough mother". The empathic attunement is found repeatedly in Winnicott's work as are descriptions of interferences with the mother's mir-roring functions that lead to the development of a "false self" by creating "a distortion in the ego" [49, 50]. However, although the environment facilit-ates an internally determined maturational process, the experiences generated by the environment are not considered to affect the processes of internaliza-tion. "The environment does not make the infant grow, nor does it deter-mine the direction of growth. The environment, when good enough, facilitates a maturational process" [49]. Kohut, on the other hand, on the basis of his observation of the various selfobject transferences, postulated a process of transmuting internalization of the environment's empathic responses that can occur not only during infancy but throughout development. Examples of this process of internalization related to the transitional object and signal anxiety have been carefully detailed by Tolpin [47].

Since our focus is on parenting, we are only summarizing the selfobject functions that appear to be responsible for the development of a vigorous, cohesive self. From the merger experiences of infancy to the mirroring that affirms the toddler's initiative and self-assertiveness, the mirroring that vali-dates the legitimacy of the rivalry and jealousy of the oedipal age child, the parent (ideally) continues to mirror affirmatively the adolescent's develop-ment; "divergences" and differences between parent and child put a particular strain on parental empathy. Parallel to these mirroring and validating experiences and combined with them are innumerable experiences in which the child is merged with the parents' (idealized) strength and power. The calm firmness of a parent's arms (or voice) as it calms the agitated child represents a selfobject function that, through repetition and optimal frustration, becomes the child's own ability to calm and soothe him- or herself. Repeated, innumerable merger experiences account for the development of the child's capacity to reduce tension and to tolerate anxiety. At later phases of development, these experiences concern themselves less with the child being merged with the parents' physical strength than with their moral strength and ideals.

The transformation of infantile grandiosity and exhibitionism into vigor, vitality, self-esteem (through phase-appropriate mirroring), and the establishment of valued ideals (through merger experiences with the idealized object) is not "completed" during the first few years of life. Self-assertive, grandiose, and exhibitionistic needs are in evidence throughout childhood, particularly during the oedipal phase of development; ideals and goals of the nuclear self become firmed up during adolescence. With physical growth, acquisition of new skills, and the tentative expression of innate talents, the child's growing self continually needs to be affirmed and firmed up by mirroring and idealized selfobject responses.

5.3 Parental self-development and parental empathy

Parenting, especially during infancy and the early years of the child's life, requires emotional resources that are not required by ordinary life stresses. Parents may be well-functioning adults in other ways, but discreet deficits in their own self-development may become manifest when they become parents. Specifically, it is the development of parental empathy in relationship to a particular child that most convincingly links parenting to self-development. The parent who is capable of parental attunement is one who developed an adult form of empathy – a capacity in which an adult man or woman can immerse him- or herself into the inner life of a child without this threatening his or her own sense of separateness and without the parent injecting his or her own needs into the interaction with the child. This is a more complicated and difficult task than it is generally acknowledged. The difficulty is related primarily to the determination of a small child's motives relative to a particular behavior. Virginia Demos [18] gives an example of a toddler approaching a dangerous object such as a pair of scissors accompanied by the various possible responses a caretaker can have to such a situation. In view of the danger that the scissors represent, the caretaker may have difficulty recognizing the child's motive in reaching for the scissors – namely, the wish to explore and to express curiosity. In other words, empathy involves the recognition of the child's motives for the behavior. Since in the case of a young child only the behavior is available for observation, it is more likely that this will be interpreted in terms of the meaning that it has for the caretaker rather than the meaning that the behavior has for the child. This is particularly true once the child's motive has been partially or completely ignored and the behavior has been responded to only in terms of its meaning to the caretaker. By the time the child becomes demanding, hits, or bites because his intent has originally been misinterpreted or ignored, an inter-action has been set into motion that precludes the possibility of recognizing and responding to the child's original motives.

Understanding and appreciation of the child's internal state has to be dis-tinguished from the manner in which a parent may respond to this state; "giving in" to a child is frequently mistaken for empathy. Parental responses can only be considered empathic when they encompass the child's "reality" above and beyond his momentary and, at times, imperative demands. Under-standing and validating the child's inner state (i.e., appreciating his wish to explore, to touch, and to feel objects in his environment) does not exclude a response by the parent that is guided by mature judgment.

Demos [18] distinguished between six possible types of responses by care-givers. She was careful in pointing out that these responses do not represent types of caregivers but rather types of perceptions, inferences, and responses that any caregiver might employ. (1) The caregiver perceives accurately and understands the child's experience and acts so that the child's positive experi-ences are prolonged and enhanced, and the child's negative experiences are reduced or brought to an end. (2) The caregiver perceives accurately and understands the child's negative experiences and acts so that the child is helped to endure them and to master them. (3) The caregiver perceives accu-rately and understands the child's positive experiences and acts so that there is a reduction in these positive affects. (4) The caregiver perceives and under-stands the child's negative experiences and acts so that the child experiences an increase in negative affects. (This may be done in a nonhostile manner.) (5) The caregiver misperceives or misunderstands some or all of the child's experiences and acts according to the misperception and misunderstanding. (6) The care-giver appears not to perceive the child and acts as if the child is not present. Demos makes it clear that no single exchange has a determining impact on the child, though "each type of exchange will produce a distinc-tive type of experience for the child and that if such experiences become a chronic characteristic of the infant-mother system, they will begin to shape the child's developing sense of self" [18].

The question is frequently asked whether or not empathy means that a state of fusion exists between subject and object. This question appears to be related to the observation that empathy, an innate capacity of the human psyche, unfolds in the early years of psychological development. And while the infant, indeed, appears to be "fused" with the adult (e.g., the infant experiences the calmness or the anxiety of the adult as if this were his own), the requirements for empathic responsiveness to the infant's needs are the opposite of fusion. Adult empathy depends on the adult's capacity to retain his own sense of separateness. Fliess [20] spoke of "trial identification" and

Schafer [44] spoke of "generative empathy" to indicate that empathy is a complex and high level of mental functioning. Norman Paul [40] is most explicit about the need for the achievement of the sense of separateness in relation to an adult, that is, in relation to parental empathy.

> An empathizer, or subject, accepts for a brief period, the object's total emotional individuality, not only his simple emotions but also his whole state of being the history of his desires, feelings, and thoughts as well as other forces and experiences that are expressed in his behavior. Empathy presupposes the existence of the object as a separate individual, entitled to his own feelings, ideas, and emotional history. The empathizer makes no judgement what the other should feel and, for brief periods, experiences these feelings as his own. The empathizer oscillates between such subjective involvement and a detached recognition of the shared feelings. Secure in his sense of self and his own emotional boundaries, the empathizer attempts to nurture a similar security in the other.
>
> (p. 340)

Kohut's view of the development of empathy, namely, that empathy is the product of the successful transformation of archaic narcissism into its most mature forms (along with other highly valued psychic capacities such as wisdom, humor, and the acceptance of one's own transience) is in keeping with Paul's emphasis on the empathizer's ability to feel "secure in his sense of self and his own emotional boundaries".

With each child, the parent's empathic capacities are tested anew. Each child "creates" his own mother and father as the parents' empathic responses become "dovetailed" to the specific needs of the particular child. Herein lies the essence of parental empathy. "The parents do not respond out of their own needs, nor do they respond in keeping with prescriptions as to how to be a good parent, but their responses are determined by the needs of the particular child at a particular time in the child's life" [37]. Some parents are able to be in empathic contact with young children readily, while others do not communicate meaningfully with their children until they are older or until the children reach adolescence [36]. Such variations in parental empathic capacities are generally nontraumatic, so long as other members in the parenting unit readily substitute for the temporarily unavailable one.

However, even under the most optimal circumstances, when adults become parents with a well consolidated self, the reliable, ongoing presence of their empathy still depends essentially on two major factors: (1) the support of their social milieu, and (2) the child's ability to affirm their parenting. From the moment that a mother becomes sensitive to her baby's cry – when she differentiates between the cry that signals hunger and the one that indicates general discomfort – she relies on her empathic capacity to perceive her infant's needs. But the mother's "motherliness," her capacity for empathic responsiveness, needs to be affirmed as well; feeding, cleaning, and handling that calms and comforts the baby promotes the integration of motherliness. An unhappy, discontent infant, unable to mirror the mother because of congenital or acquired disability, interferes with the integration of motherliness and with the mother's ability to be empathic over prolonged periods of time.

Impaired babies may elicit extremes in caretaker responsiveness from over-protectiveness and oversolicitousness to overt to covert rejection. Contradictory responses may occur in the same caretaker. Because of the chronic strain related to the care of an impaired baby, there are expectable lapses in the caretaker's empathy; in the empathic caretaker this creates guilt and shame that sets the stage for increased protectiveness.

In considering the impact of the impaired infant on the caretaker, we are not only referring to the cases of grossly defective or handicapped infants in which parental responsiveness is usually fairly clear-cut   namely, either increased parental compassion, love, and tolerance or obvious signs of rejection. The problem is more complicated in relationship to subtle, subliminal impairments in a child without demonstrable clinical findings. These infants, for lack of a definitive diagnosis, have been considered to be minimally brain damaged or to have immature central nervous systems. These are infants whose subtle neurological impairments interfere with the execution and mastery of their daily routines (e.g., frequent vomiting with eating, sensitivity to noise and general irritability with sleep, poor motor coordination with the phase appropriate development of speech and locomotion). The parent, unable to feel effective in the care of the child, does not feel affirmed and experiences increasing frustration; a slow erosion of his or her empathic capacities may follow.

What needs to be emphasized is that this feedback mechanism is not restricted to infancy. The need for adequate mirroring of the parent by the child continues throughout the parents' life and becomes of particular importance to the parent with grown children. Children who have successfully mastered their various developmental tasks affirm the parents in their parenting ability and contribute to the enhancement and esteem of their adult self. The reverse is true as well: Children, who, for whatever reason, encounter difficulties in the course of their lifetime, affect their parents self-esteem to various degrees.

The parents' expectable need for affirmation of their parenting is related to the observation made by Freud: Parental love, at its roots, is "narcissistic love" [21]. It is the parent's selfobject tie (narcissistic investment) to the child that assures adequate parental care, and it is the failure of such a tie to develop that accounts for abandonment (e.g., discarding the newborn into a trash can), infanticide, or gross physical neglect.

The close tie that we are establishing between the development of the self (the transformation of archaic narcissism into its adult form, specifically into an adult form of empathy) and parenting is a departure from Benedek's conceptualization of parenting being primarily dependent on the parents' identification with their own parents. The central aspect of Benedek's [8] theory of motherliness is a double identification, one in which the mother's identification with her own mother becomes reactivated when she becomes a mother herself. As the mother identifies with the baby's regressive needs, she becomes both (i.e., her mother who has cared for her and her baby who is the recipient of this care). This concept of double identification has been useful to the clinician for the understanding of the various expressions of maternal dysfunctions. For example, when mothers make a conscious effort to care for their babies differently from the way they experienced their own mother's care, they may find that powerful unconscious identifications with their own mother interfere with their most avid conscious intent.

As useful as Benedek's theory of double identification has been, the theory has limitations as an explanatory principle both for relatively conflict-free as well as pathological forms of parenting. Identification would indicate a fixed, predictable pattern in parental responsiveness and could not account for the changes that clinicians regularly observe in parents; parents, as adults and as parents, continue to grow and develop in relationship to the same child as well as in relationship to their various children. For this reason, Brody [14] questioned the usefulness of Benedek's "identification theory" and suggested that empathy may be a better concept than identification to describe ongoing, flexible, maternal behavior. Brody's view was supported by Parens, who suggested that parenthood may not be best conceptualized as the final culmination of the psychosexual line of development. Rather, it should be considered as part of the total personality development and could best be understood as part of "the line of development pertaining to the concept of the self" [39]. As we have already indicated, we agree with this view and add that we consider parenting as one of the most important challenges to the consolidation and esteem of the adult's self. The demands of parenting will either prove to be disorganizing and fragmenting to a poorly consolidated adult self or will constitute a challenge that will bring about an enrichment and refinement to the self similar to that provided by other creative and artistic endeavors. It is in this context that we are reminded of Erikson's statement that "generativity which is concerned with new beings as well as new products and new ideas and which, as a link between the generations, is as indispensable for the renewal of the adult generations own life as it is for that of the next generation" [19].

A further question regarding the identification theory of parenting is related to the inevitability of repetition-the generation-to-generation transfer of inadequate parenting. For example, when the observation is made that abusive parents have been abused children, this does not mean that all parents who have been abused as children become abusive parents. The process that evolves between parents and children and the parents' self-development as it continues throughout their adult life is an intricate and complex process and contradicts a fixed pattern that is assumed by the theory of early identifications.

Viewing the evolution of parenting as integral to self-development shifts the emphasis from the inevitability of repetition and helps instead to conceptualize the way parenting itself provides an opportunity for furthering the development of the adult self. This is in keeping with Benedek's view that parenthood is a developmental phase [9] or rather, a developmental process [14], which implies a structural rather than simply a behavioral change. As we have indicated earlier, this developmental process is made possible because of the narcissistic investment that parents have in their children. While it is this narcissistic investment in the child that assures adequate parental care, it is also the narcissistic nature of the parent-child tie that makes parenting a vulnerable adult function and accounts for its various forms of pathology.

5.4 Parental dysfunctions: diagnosis and treatment

In the clinical situation, psychotherapists are rarely consulted because of parental dysfunctions; their diagnosis and treatment becomes important when parents bring their already symptomatic children to a psychotherapist.

By the time parents seek professional help, they have recognized that they have been caught in an ever-tightening web of pathological interactions with their symptomatic child. Not understanding the nature, or rather the meaning, of the child's behavior, they react to it with anger and disappointment, which in turn create new problems that quickly cover up or accentuate the original difficulties. There occurs a "layering" of interactions between the various members of the family over time; the parents may become increasingly more rigid and punitive or appeasing and placating as they attempt to deal with the child's symptomatic behavior. Such parental attitudes are secondary: They are responses to the child's symptoms and should not be considered to be the cause of the child's original difficulties. What the professional sees at the time of the diagnostic assessment is the end product of years of pathological interactions that have had serious consequences not only for the child's development but for the parent's parenting capacities as well.

Parental dysfunctions are difficult to diagnose unless they take overt forms such as physical or sexual abuse, neglect, or abandonment. Features of parenting that we have been describing are frequently silent and usually subtle such as the proud gleam in the caretaker's eye or the tone in his or her voice. Failures in these subtle but active parental responses easily elude the clinician and are never reported because they are, more often than not, unconscious to the parents themselves. Nor are these observations readily available to the child. Caretakers, who in all other respects are attentive, may still not be able to perceive and respond to the child's developmentally determined narcissistic needs. Also, empathic failures may be "hidden" behind claims of love and material indulgences. Under these circumstances, the child finds himself emotionally trapped: He experiences his rage at the caretakers as unfounded. These children may use their own body to inflict pain on those, who, because of their inability to comprehend and respond empathically, have emotionally abandoned them. These are children who attempt or threaten to commit suicide or whose self-destructive behavior may take covert forms such as reckless driving, indiscriminate use of drugs, and running away. The self-destructive behavior represents both the expression of revenge as well as an expression of the inadequate narcissistic investment of the body: their body is not worth saving. The tragedy of this particular outcome of parental dysfunctions is that the child's rage at the parent remains largely unconscious or unacceptable, and his despair is compounded by guilt as the self-destructive behavior is considered "unexplainable." The caretaker, sensitive to the element of revenge but not able to perceive the child's pain, may experience the child's self-destructive behavior as an indictment against him- or herself.

Kohut warned that "the complexity of the pathogenic interplay between parent and child and the limitless varieties of it defy the attempt of a comprehensive description" [27]. However, in reconstructing the genesis of his patient's psychopathology, he described a spectrum of parental disturbances that "may extend from mild narcissistic fixations to latent or overt psychosis", and it was his impression that "a specific type of covert psychosis in a parent tends to produce broader and deeper fixations in the narcissistic and especially in the prenarcissistic (autoerotic) realm than does overt psychosis." Overt psychosis in the primary caretaker has its own pathogenic impact on a child. The child "adapts" to the often bizarre, frightening behavior, the repeated need for hospitalizations, and the particularly dulling effects of many of the antipsychotic medications in such a way that no symptoms may be manifested in childhood but only later in life. However, the fact that the parental disturbance is overt appears to protect the child from the kinds of internal compromises that children whose parents suffer from various degrees of discreet forms of self-pathology have to make. In the case of an overt disturbance of a caretaker, the child's own perceptions are more clearly validated and he or she can turn more freely to other members in the parenting unit to provide the developmentally crucial selfobject responses. This assures the child of adequate consolidation of his self and the capacity to be resilient to the behavior of the disturbed caretaker.

In a child therapist's everyday practice, the largest group of dysfunctional caretakers suffer from relatively discreet forms of self-pathology. These are caretakers, who, because of self-absorption, are not available to perceive their children's states of mind and who frequently project their own moods into their emotional environments. It is also the caretaker with the discreet forms of self-deficit who may selectively "overrespond" to certain aspects of the child's personality – aspects more in keeping with his or her expectations for self-enhancement than in keeping with the child's own talents and temperament.

In diagnosing, the degree and nature of self-disorder that underlie the various forms of parental dysfunctions, it is useful to distinguish between caretakers who emotionally distance themselves from the child whom they can no longer fit into their self-regulatory system (especially when another child has a more successful fit) from those who insist on remaining in the center of the child's universe. This latter group of parents unconsciously create a sense of responsibility in their child for their own self-cohesion and/or for the maintenance of their own self-esteem.

Parents who "use" their children either to maintain self-cohesion or self-esteem are particularly vulnerable to rage reactions since the child is likely to frustrate their infantile, now highly intensified, selfobject needs. This explains the frequently violent attacks with which these children may be physically or verbally abused.

In relationship to physical child abuse, we found the work of Steele [45] particularly illuminating because this author had consistently used an empathic approach in his study of the child-abusing caretaker. In the psychological profiles he had sketched, we recognize people whose self-disorder had become manifest in relationship to the demand that parenthood had made on them. Steele's data support our thesis that failures in parenting are most likely to occur when parents use their children to fill their own inner emptiness or to bolster their own shaky self-esteem. The description of "the attack," the abusive act itself, helps us appreciate the imperative nature of the parent's unconscious demand to have the infant (or child) meet the caretaker's selfobject needs of the moment. The following sequence tells the story clearly. The caretaker approaches the child with a genuine intent to care for him. However, this is always accompanied by a deep, hidden yearning for the infant to respond in a highly specific way. When the infant fails to respond according to these expectations "a harsh, authoritative demand for the infant's correct response, supported by a sense of parental rightness, follows" [45]. Only when we take the imperative need for the fulfillment of the parent's selfobject need into consideration can we fully appreciate why the infant's failure to smile or otherwise express his or her appreciation for the parent's ministrations is experienced by the parent as rejection – a severe form of narcissistic injury. Steele makes it very clear that these are not ordinary, expectable parental displeasures that "can be aroused if the baby is temperamentally either very active or passive when the opposite type was hoped for." Rather, "the common denominator in the situation where abuse occurs is the innocent infant's failure to meet exaggerated, unyielding parental need" [45].

The recognition of the child-abusing caretaker as one who suffers from a form of self-pathology in which the child is expected to be responsive to an "exaggerated, unyielding parental need" can be distinguished from the caretaker who had failed to develop a selfobject tie with the child altogether. The latter form of parental dysfunction is expressed in abandonment or in chronic physical and emotional neglect. It is not the subject of this chapter to elaborate on the difference in the form that the child's psychopathology may take when he or she experiences chronic neglect rather than periodic and harsh abuse. Suffice it to say that chronic indifference is likely to result in various forms of childhood depression, low self-esteem, and lack of initiative; children who have been abused physically may be subservient to the abusing caretaker but are likely to become aggressive and provocative with younger children and/or animals.

More often than not, children perceive the parent's anxiety in relation to the parent's self-cohesion and/or self-esteem and readily comply with parental expectations at the expense of their own progressive development. This compliance is the function of the imperative developmental need to retain contact with the selfobject milieu. Winnicott called this particular form of adaptation an "impingement" on the child's psyche. "If reacting to impingements is the pattern of the infant's life, then there is a serious interference with the natural tendency that exists in the infant to become an integrated unit, able to continue to have a self with a past, present, and future" [49]. The reference here to impingements as patterns is of importance, indicating that impingements also occur with "good-enough" mothering but create distortions in the ego when they become regular or sustained and thereby constitute patterns.

In the same way that a parent may "impinge" only on certain areas of the child's development, emotional abandonment may also be restricted to a particular segment of the child's personality. Parents may affirm selectively certain of the child's physical or intellectual attributes. But as far as the child is concerned, such arbitrarily selective affirmation may be experienced as a parental failure to validate other aspects of the developing self – that is, an outright rejection of his or her total self. In his reconstructions of the wholesome development of the self, Kohut emphasized the mirroring selfobject's response to the "total self" of the infant or child as opposed to his or her isolated bodily or mental functions. A response to the whole child at first enhances the establishment of the cohesiveness of the self, and later on it contributes to the maintenance of this recently acquired and, therefore, still precarious unity of the self. "The mother's exultant response to the total child (calling him by name as she enjoys his presence and activity) supports ... the growth of the self experience as a physical and mental unit which has cohesiveness in space and continuity in time" [27]. In a clinical example Kohut illustrates the untoward results of an arbitrarily or inappropriately selective maternal response to a body part or behavioral detail, which not only detracts attention from the child's total self, his central wish, or purpose of the moment, but is experienced by the child as a serious rejection of his whole being. "When Mr. B. would tell his mother exuberantly about some achievement or experience, she seemed not only to be cold or inattentive but, instead of responding to him and the event that he was describing, would suddenly remark critically about a detail of his appearance or current behavior: 'Don't move your hands while you are talking!' This reaction must have been experienced by the son not only as a rejection of the particular display for which he needed a confirming response but also as an active destruction of the cohesiveness of his self experience (by shifting attention to apart of his body) just at the most vulnerable moment when he was offering his total self for approval" [27]. For the child, to feel connected with and responded to by the parent is very important for survival. For this reason, infants and young children "adapt" early to parental attitudes, restrictions, and expectations that may stunt, distort, or otherwise compromise the child's developing self.

In addition to considering the various forms of self-pathology that facilitate the clinician's understanding of parental dysfunctions, it is also important to recognize how a particular developmental phase may become stressful to a particular caretaker. For this reason, we shall describe clinical situations of parental dysfunctions that correspond to various developmental phases in the child.

5.5 Clinical examples

In terms of childhood and adult psychopathology, no other developmental phase appears to be as heavily implicated as the toddler years. Mahler, in her extensive work with toddlers and their mothers, noted that many mothers at this time "make a sharp turnabout in the overall quality of their maternal care in response to maturational events" [35]. Mahler's explanation for this sudden change in the mother's responsiveness rests on her observation that some mothers are unable to promote separation and individuation because of their own need to retain symbiotic fusion with the child. This need for symbiosis, in turn, she said, was determined by the fact that the baby frequently represented a part of the mother's body, specifically the phallus. "In our study ... we sometimes see, in the way some of the mothers talk about the baby's body, how they hold and handle it, that the infant has the meaning of an illusory phallus for the mother." In addition to this more general meaning, each child has a more "specific meaning for the mother, according to the general and the specific fantasy connected with each child by that mother" [34].

What Mahler described here are instances in which the baby is perceived as part (or rather the missing part) of the mother's body. Physical separation under these circumstances becomes intolerable because the toddler-age child will no longer comply with the mother's wish to be held and be handled in such a way as to help the mother maintain her fantasied illusion that he or she is part of her body. Considering that such "misuse" or "misperception" of the baby may occur in a broader psychological context, we conclude that a mother who "makes a sharp turnabout" in her mothering when her baby becomes a toddler is not necessarily responding to the threat of physical separation, but rather to the baby's new demands on her, which fails to complete or enhance the mother's self in the manner in which this was possible in relationship to a younger infant.

In our view, there are various fundamental reasons that may explain why the toddler years are so heavily implicated in childhood psychopathology. The toddler's increasing self-assertiveness and autonomy as well as a more forceful introduction of individual characteristics, especially temperament, bring new qualities into the "interactive regulatory system" [43]. A new level of the infant's self-organization requires something from the environment that is very different from that of the crib infant. From the emphasis on the establishment on homeostasis in the first year of life, for which the clues may not have been easy to pick up by the environment but which, on the whole, could still be readily "accommodated" into the parent's own self-regulatory system, the toddler "demands" recognition and admiration for his or her initiative, which may dramatically confront the parent's own purposes and values. A similar form of "confrontation," though obviously on a different level of development, occurs during adolescence.

What needs to be reemphasized here is that selfobject responses, such as the validation of the child's unique way of asserting him- or herself, are active parental responses. In other words, what may function as a potentially pathogenic agent is not only the presence of an untoward response to the toddler's self-assertiveness but the *absence of a developmentally needed active response* such as the overt and enthusiastic expression of joy.

The toddler years are prime times for the experience of omnipotence and exhibitionism. Toddlers experience themselves in the center of the universe; they are now filled with a sense of initiative and healthy vigor. They want those around them to see, recognize, and acknowledge their intoxicating sense of what they have discovered to be their own powers and abilities. To an environment that is fearful of losing its control over, the toddler's developmentally exaggerated sense of power, this behavior will be threatening. Under these circumstances, the environment anxiously attempts to reinforce its control, battles ensue, and a child's self-assertion disintegrates into the aimless and frequently destructive form of aggression. Children who respond to the increased control with aggression appear to maintain their self-assertiveness to a greater degree than those who give up on their initiative and become withdrawn and apathetic. This latter group of children is more likely to suffer from chronic narcissistic rage that brings about the character disorders that, at a later date, are recognized for their masochistic, paranoid, or depressive features. In other words, "the divergence" [42] or the "sharp turnabout" [35] that so commonly occurs between the toddler and his or her emotional environment may result in overt symptoms during childhood, or this divergence may remain latent and lead to some form of self-disorder later in life. In terms of overt symptoms, we witness an increase in the intensity of separation anxiety; the toddler becomes clingy and whiny and develops nightmares and other forms of sleep disturbances. Tolpin and Kohut [48] maintain that the usual childhood anxieties (e.g., fear of the dark, noise, animals, and robbers or the development of compulsive rituals) are the manifestations of "disintegration" and "depletion" anxiety created by the child feeling "unplugged" from the life-sustaining connection with his or her primary selfobject.

The following clinical example shall demonstrate a form of parental dysfunction in which the child's progressive development interfered with the mother's precariously maintained self-esteem regulation. Once the child became symptomatic, further complications ensued. The clinical example shall also permit the discussion of the implications for treatment when the nature of the parental dysfunctions are given primary consideration in the treatment of the child.

Martin and his parents

Martin was 4 years old when he was brought by his parents to a therapist, a woman, who was trained as a child analyst. The parents complained that the child was still enuretic and that in nursery school he was shy and withdrawn. This was in contrast to his provocative and "rebellious" behavior at home, especially in relationship to his mother.

Martin was the oldest of two children. His mother had him when she was 32 years old. Prior to her pregnancy she had several jobs, but none satisfied her. She described her efforts in this respect (as well as her various attempts to complete her education) as failures because of her lack of self-confidence.

The first year after Martin's birth was "blissful." Martin was a bright and responsive baby. However, battles between mother and son began in the child's second year of life; he proved to be "hard to train," and at the time of referral he was still enuretic. The father had little to do with Martin. As a young aspiring professional, he spent long hours in his office. When Martin was 2, the father became aware of the struggles between mother and son and wanted to make himself available to them. However, the mother asked that the father leave them alone and insisted that raising Martin was to be her "career."

The first two diagnostic interviews revealed an anxious little boy who was shy and very hard to engage. The therapist assessed the child as one who had "a cohesive self" with a firm hold on his object world and whose symptoms, on the basis of his play activities and associations, could be related to "phallic conflicts emanating from his emerging sexuality, castration fears, and the wish and fear to exhibit his penis and his body." Because the symptoms could be related to a structural neurotic conflict and were considered to be precipitated by the birth of his sister whom his mother "adored," the recommendation was for the child to enter psychoanalysis and for his parents to see a social worker occasionally. This latter decision was based on the fact that the parents appeared to have been "well-intended, intelligent people who were eager to cooperate in their son's treatment."

The parents agreed to the recommendation and the first six months of analysis confirmed the therapist's predictions: the child had improved considerably, except for his enuresis. The changes were most pronounced in the therapist's office. From a shy, withdrawn child, Martin changed to a vigorous and self-assertive one. The changes, the therapist felt, were directly related to her vigorous interpretations of the child's sexual and exhibitionistic wishes and his castration fears.

However, as the child improved, the mother, rather than being pleased, appeared to become increasingly more unhappy. She began to focus on Martin's enuresis and exposed the child to a series of painful physical examinations that resulted in the diagnosis of "a small urethral meatus." Only because of the therapist's interventions was surgery avoided.

At this time the parents were referred for treatment to their own therapists, and the mother spoke of Martin in extremely negative terms. In response, the therapist made great efforts to "correct" this "distorted perception" because she herself viewed Martin as a lively and engaging boy. The therapist was also "repelled" by the mother's "confession" that in spite of her friends' and doctor's advice not to yell at Martin when he wet his pants, she could not do otherwise. As the therapist reinforced the advice previously given to the mother, and as she continued to correct the mother's "distorted perception" of the child, the mother's anger increased and she abruptly terminated her own and the boy's treatment. The father continued to see the social worker for a while but he felt increasingly more helpless to do anything about the situation, and eventually he, too, discontinued treatment.

Treatment implications

In reviewing the treatment of this child and his parents, we are not questioning the theoretical frame of reference that had guided the analyst in her interpretations of the child's fantasies and the meaning of his play activities; the child responded favorably to the therapist's interpretations of his sexual wishes and castration fears and he became vigorous and self-assertive with her. Our focus, instead, is on the treatment of the parents and the therapist's failure to have diagnosed and properly treated the self-disorder that affected the mother's parenting in the second year of the child's life. We believe that it was this that was responsible for the mother removing the child from treatment; her anger at Martin who so blatantly exposed her "inadequacy" increased with his improvement, and she had to find some explanation, other than a psychological one, for his problems.

The mother's initial insistence that the father should not participate in the child's care, that caring for him was to be her career, indicates the importance it had for the mother to experience herself as a competent, successful parent. This had particular importance to her in light of her deep sense of inadequacy in other areas of her life; the child was to help her develop a sense of perfection about herself. Martin did this as an infant but not as a toddler. The introduction of his lively temperament into "the interactive system" tested the limits of her empathic capacity. Once Martin failed to confirm the mother in the perfection of her motherliness, she increased her efforts to reestablish control over him. This resulted in the child's self-assertion degenerating into hostility and he became symptomatic, which further undermined the mother's self-esteem. When the mother insisted on a physical exploration of Martin's enuresis, she was not only trying to restitute her self-esteem but, through the painful procedure, she was also "punishing" the child for having failed her.

The importance of making the child's emotional environment an active partner in the treatment process is directly related to our use of the model of the self-selfobject unit in organizing our data and in planning the child's treatment. The child's inner world (i.e., developmental events, anxieties, and symptoms) cannot be fully understood without the environment that shapes and continually affects this intrapsychic reality. The improvement that a young child achieves in the therapist's office cannot be simply "transferred" to the home – certainly not when the parents cannot respond to the symptomatic child with the same empathic understanding as the therapist.

But how is the therapist to help a parent develop empathy toward his or her symptomatic child? We believe that a process that enhances parental empathy can be set into motion if the therapist also encompasses empathically the parents' psychic reality. While it is true that in order to know how the child experiences the parent subjectively the therapist has to immerse him- or herself empathically into the inner world of the child, such an immersion into the child's inner world does not exclude the therapist from empathically encompassing the psychic reality of the parents as well. The therapist is not asked to take sides: He or she is asked to understand and to explain.

However, in the treatment of children, this particular caveat of not taking sides appears to be particularly difficult to observe. Listening to case conferences in which families and their troubled children are being discussed, it appears to be extremely difficult for the professional not to create or reinforce guilt in the parents for their children's emotional difficulties. From the extreme of "parentectomy," the forceful separation of parent and child, to the recommendation that the parents have treatment for themselves, without which their child cannot be helped, parents are frequently treated by professionals primarily as people who can only create problems but who cannot remedy them. However, because we consider the parents' empathic responsiveness to the troubled child as one of the crucial therapeutic agents, we would suggest that therapists of children of all ages, but certainly those of young children, focus their attention on the specific features in the parents' personalities that have made the parenting of this particular child, at this particular time in the child's and the parents' lives, difficult for them. Such an approach to treatment requires that the therapist fully appreciate the child's intrapsychic state and his or her vulnerabilities, anxieties, and defenses, and, at the same time, become acquainted with the source of the parents' limitations for empathic responsiveness to a child who is manifesting various disturbing symptoms to the environment.

The parents' fear of "exposing" themselves to a professional appears to be justified. In the case of Martin's mother, for example, instead of understanding the mother's reason for viewing her child as "bad," the therapist attempted to correct this perception. Parental dysfunctions are symptoms that require exploration, understanding, and explanation as do other psychological symptoms. Martin's mother needed to find out why she felt bad about the child and what had turned this originally blissful relationship into such a difficult one. When the therapist does not appreciate the narcissistic mortification that parents experience for having a troubled child and when the parents feel further reduced in their self-esteem because they are not included into the therapeutic effort, it is then that they are most likely to remove the child from treatment or look for an explanation other than the psychological one for the child's difficulties.

When we consider the consequences of the caretaker's need to control the child's phase-appropriate curiosity, motility, and self-assertion, it is also important to recognize that, in relationship to this particular caretaker, the child has also been deprived of the affirmative responses that are essential to this phase of his development. Martin could have received these from his father who, however, could not meaningfully interact with him because of the mother's insistence that she be the only one responsible for his care. The result was that a structural deficit became manifest; in nursery school Martin was shy and withdrawn and he lacked vigor and lively interest in his surroundings.

A child such as Martin is likely to acquire necessary skills and may continue to develop but remains detached and only marginally involved with people and events around him. Greenspan [23] makes a similar point in relationship to the infant in whom the major developmental task is the establishment and maintenance of homeostasis. The optimal capacity for homeostasis, he says, involves the integration of developmentally facilitating life experiences in the fullest sense. It is this that assures the initiation of human relationships and interest in the environment. In other words, there is a qualitative difference between the infant who has the capacity to interact with his or her environment when homeostasis is assured by the presence of a calming "other" and the infant who has to "sacrifice" the optimal state of alertness and engagement in order to remain calm.

Bobby and his parents

A brief discussion of the case reported by Burlingham and colleagues [16] should further support our thesis that the successful treatment of a child, especially that of a young child, requires that the child's emotional milieu be helped to develop the capacity to respond empathically to the symptomatic child, which would make the continuation of the child's development within the same regulative system possible.

As with the treatment of Martin, Bobby, too, was taken into analysis because he appeared to have "a good potential for improvement or even complete recovery." However, in spite of the mother's conscious efforts to cooperate in the treatment, the child's symptoms could not be fully understood until the mother was taken into analysis herself where her "unconscious fantasies and attitudes" could be explored.

This was a simultaneous analysis of mother and son. The two treatment processes, however, were kept carefully separated so as to keep "the two therapists independent and uninfluenced by the material of the other partner"; the two analysts were instructed not to communicate with each other. The mother may not have been expected to be able to appreciate the motives of the child's behavior but, importantly, the father's help was not enlisted in this effort. Bobby, like Martin, did not display any of the behavior problems related to eating and the regulation of his bowel habits with his father although he did with his mother. It would appear that the resiliency that was noted in Bobby was related to an adequate and most likely compensatory structuralization of his psyche in which the father, rather than the mother, functioned as an empathically responsive, mirroring selfobject.

Bobby's symptoms were identical to the mother's childhood symptoms, especially those concerning the withholding of feces. The authors reported that the mother, as a child, forced her own mother to remain with her during defecation: "to keep her feces inside came to represent only means to get attention and not to feel lonely" [16]. Now, as a mother, she could not tolerate being separated from Bobby. Her need to infantilize the child and thereby keep him close to her, was interpreted as "proof of her hate for her child and her death wishes against him. When the child showed pleasure in being without her, he symbolized her own mother who had withdrawn from her" [16].

We are questioning the interpretation of the mother's separation anxiety as "proof of her hate for her child." Based on the mother's analytic material, the mother's need for the child's presence is a direct continuation of her efforts to control her own mother. She hated the child most intensely when she was not successful in this effort (i.e., "when the child showed pleasure in being without her" [16]). The rage reaction here is secondary to the frustration that the mother experienced when she could not control the responses of the selfobject child. This conceptualization affects the interpretive process. Rather than interpreting the mother's separation anxiety as the expression of her hate and death wishes toward the child, the rage would have to be interpreted as secondary to her efforts to control the child in order to feel affirmed by him. The mother could only feel affirmed if she could experience herself as the only one to whom the child responded with pleasure.

This clinical report of a simultaneous analysis of mother and child is of significance for our thesis because it confirms Kohut's (re)constructions [27] regarding the pathogenesis of failures in parental empathy. According to Burlingham [16], "Seen from the point of view of this child's analysis, we would say that, through his behavior, Bobby forced the mother to react toward him as she did. Seen from the aspect of the mother's analysis, Bobby's behavior takes on a different connotation. There is, in the mother's analytic material, ample evidence that in handling the child's feeding situation she was herself under the domination of powerful unconscious fantasies which determined her attitude. In this light the child's behavior will be seen as a reaction to the mother's provocation." However, if the two analysts could not communicate in order to remain "independent and uninfluenced by the material of the other partner," the child's analyst could not benefit from this insight and the child's behavior would be interpreted, as indeed it was, as an expression of his anal ambivalence, his death wishes, and sexual wishes toward his mother. The mother's treatment, in turn, could not benefit from the recognition that it was the mother's need to keep herself in the center of the child's universe that had perpetuated the child's psychopathology.

We have elaborated on the case of Bobby for several reasons. Along with Martin's case, Bobby's case, too, demonstrates many of the problems that are related to parental dysfunctions and their treatment. Both clinical examples highlighted the importance of involving the child's emotional environment in the treatment process in a specific way namely, by recognizing and interpreting the specific functions that the child is serving in the parent's psychic life.

These two clinical examples also demonstrate the usefulness of the concept of the parenting unit. For both boys, the fathers apparently had fulfilled certain basic selfobject functions so that when away from their mothers, they could function adequately. Bobby's treatment team had not taken advantage of this circumstance; Martin's treatment team did but without success. We are suggesting that the successful treatment of a child is best assured when available resources are mobilized in addition to the attention given to the pathological interaction with one member of the parenting unit. The importance of such an involvement in the treatment process of members of the parenting unit who are capable of responding to the child empathically is related to the way in which we conceptualize the building up of psychological structures within the empathically responsive selfobject milieu. For a young child, everyday experiences (e.g., being fed, put to bed, sent off to school) are of "structure building" significance. When members of a parenting unit "step in" to provide the child with "average expectable" responsiveness, they not only facilitate the disengagement from a pathological enmeshment with one of its members, but they are, at the same time, providing selfobject functions that facilitate the development of compensatory structures rather than primarily defensive ones.[4] Obviously, this is only possible if the member of the parenting unit who is pathologically involved with the child permits others to participate in the child's care. Martin's father, for example, was very much aware of the importance that his emotional presence had for the child. But the mother, because of her own imperative need to establish her credentials as a mother, could not allow the father to establish a meaningful contact with the boy.

The significance of the emotional presence of caretakers of both genders in the development of children of both sexes has been repeatedly asserted [1, 23, 25]. The father or another male in the parenting unit may be available as a primary selfobject when the mother's self-pathology prevents her from being optimally responsive to the infant's merger and mirroring needs. This not only provides an opportunity for the building up of compensatory psychic structures, but the child can also experience the father as strong (independent of the mother) and therefore idealizable. The developmental significance of the boy's idealization of his father can be derived from the reconstruction of transferences of adult patients as well as from the treatment of boys whose fathers have been out of the home in the early years of the child's life or emotionally not available to them [25, 29, 38].

In order to discuss further the specific importance that the idealization of the same sex parent has for a child's development, we have selected the case of a boy who was raised by his mother and who became symptomatic after a man had moved into their home. The case shall also illustrate the challenges that are faced by single parents and how "impingements" or compromises to the child's self-development that occur earlier in life may be responsible for symptoms at a later developmental phase.

Dean and his mother

Dean was 9 years old when he and his mother came to the clinic. The mother complained of a major change in Dean's personality since her lover, Mr. Hillard, had moved into their home and the two had decided to get married. Dean, who up until now had been a fairly even-tempered and pleasant child, had become sullen and rebellious. His school work deteriorated rapidly and he refused to go to school on a number of occasions.

Dean was an illegitimate child. His mother was 17 years old when she became pregnant, and by then she had a history of alcohol and drug abuse. However, during her pregnancy she did not drink or smoke and after delivery she surprised her welfare worker with the natural competence with which she cared for the baby. The first two years the mother devoted herself completely to the care of the child. She took good care of him and their small apartment. When Dean was about 2 years old, mother took a job as a janitor in an office building. This was a night job and she took Dean with her; the child made himself at home in this environment and would easily fall asleep on one of the sofas available in these offices. With her work, mother resumed some of her drinking. She took Dean to the bar with her and the patrons there took to the bright-eyed youngster; they would take him on their laps and play with him. He was definitely the center of attention. Dean "entertained" these people to his mother's great delight. By the time Dean was 6 years old, his acting skills were considerable and his mother enrolled him in a special school where he could study acting. He liked school and did well in all his subjects but particularly in acting, securing parts in school plays and some TV commercials for which he was paid. The only thing that indicated that not all was well was Dean's shoplifting behavior. He took small items his mother could easily have afforded. Otherwise, his engaging manner and polite behavior did not reveal that the child was suffering from any form of childhood emotional disorder.

However, this attitude and behavior changed rather drastically when, for the first time in his life, a man moved into their small apartment. Not only had Dean's disposition changed, but so did his mother's: she demanded that he be nice to the man who wanted to marry her. Mr. Hillard, too, who at first took kindly to the child, began to demand that Dean show him respect by calling him "Daddy." Dean refused, insisting that since this man was not his father, he should not have to call him that. Violent fights ensued in which Dean felt betrayed by his mother, who consistently belittled and challenged him. After he ran away from home several times and threatened suicide, he was placed by the court into a group home. Here he did somewhat better, but he remained suicidal and refused to return home and to his previous school.

The most impressive feature of the joint interview with mother and son was the total absence of the mother's empathy in relation to the child's predicament. Whatever the child's motives were for feeling and behaving the way he did, the mother could not appreciate this; she could not understand why Dean wouldn't do something that was so important to her like he always did. In his own treatment, Dean spoke earnestly about suicide; the loss of interest in acting was the first sign of his depression. Acting was the major connection between him and his mother. He was no longer sure if it was he himself who wanted to go to this special school or whether it was his mother who wanted him to go into acting and he had done so only to keep her happy.

Treatment implications

What emerged in the treatment of this very articulate little boy was a picture we see rather frequently in children who, after relatively adequate early nurturing during the first two years of life, "discover" a particular mode of behavior that secures for them the echoing and approving responses of their environment, which permits the consolidation of their self-structures at least in a narrow area. But in the case of Dean, as in children similar to him, the growing self remained vulnerable to traumatic disappointments because its consolidation was only partial and related rather rigidly to one particular segment of his personality. This segment, importantly, was one that established the connection between the child and his mother and assured adequate selfobject responsiveness from her as well as from the people at the bar.

From the time of conception, Dean fulfilled important selfobject functions for his mother. Being able to carry and give birth to a child made her feel, for the first time in her life, that she was a worthwhile human being. However, once she went back to work and began to drink again, her responsiveness to him became capricious and dependent on how well Dean was able to please her. Dean, with the hyperalertness of a child who had to extract from the environment what he needed for his emotional survival, was able to establish a workable "fit" with his mother. The mother's lack of empathy became obvious only when the demand on Dean for adaptation exceeded his psychological reserves: the child was not prepared to deal with feelings of rivalry, jealousy, and possessiveness. Because of the inadequate consolidation of his self, he experienced profound despair, disintegration anxiety, and a serious suicidal intent.

The aim of treatment was to enable the child to experience the affects that this triangular relationship demanded of him. This treatment approach was based on a self-psychological perspective on the Oedipus complex – a perspective according to which "the presence of a firm self is a precondition for the experience of the Oedipus complex. Unless the child sees himself as a delimited, abiding, independent center of initiative, he is unable to experience the object-instinctual desires that lead to the conflicts and secondary adaptations of the oedipal period" [28]. When such a self-state is not yet attained, the impact of the oedipal affects and conflicts is of a very different experiential quality. "Any person afflicted with serious threats to the continuity, the consolidation, the firmness of the self will experience the Oedipus complex, despite its anxieties and conflicts, as a joyfully accepted reality" [28]. Self psychology emphasizes thus the positive aspects of the oedipal experience – positive features that are acquired not as a result of the resolution of the Oedipus complex, but "as a primary, intrinsic aspect of the experience itself" [28].

Dean's individual treatment began when he was still in the group home. The treatment plan included regular meetings with his mother and Mr. Hillard so that the therapist could understand them and help them understand the child in depth. In the meetings with mother and Mr. Hillard, the mother soon focused on her own childhood, especially on her adolescence when she began to drink and when she became pregnant with Dean. The mother, crying most of the time, spoke of the emptiness she felt during those years, how easy it was for her to find relief in alcohol, and how, for the first time in her life, she felt she did something worthwhile when she gave birth to her child. She felt that Dean had "cured" her; she did not need to drink – he filled her up with his smile and by being such a good baby. She did not seriously consider marriage until she met Mr. Hillard who, somewhat older than herself, was tender and affectionate toward her. And now she felt betrayed and let down by the child as he appeared to block her in her effort to make a better life for both of them.

We will not detail this family's treatment here further but wish to emphasize that it was crucial for Dean's recovery to mobilize the mother's empathy in relation to his predicament. This occurred by the therapist's appreciation of the mother's need to have Dean be responsive to her now as he had been in the past. By linking the mother's need for the child's responses to her to the emotional deprivation of her childhood, the mother was able to recognize that Dean's behavior was not in defiance of her; rather, it expressed the child's fear that unless he is the only one who can please her, he will lose her altogether. For Dean, the question was, "Up until now I was the one who made mother happy; will she still be there for me once someone else cares for her?"

Once Dean returned home, he and his stepfather got along very well. Though Dean did not call him "Dad," he enjoyed the many masculine activities that Mr. Hillard and he shared. He refused to return to the acting school and engaged in other mildly rebellious behavior. With the child's development fairly securely on its way, it was the mother who needed to continue her individual treatment.

In relation to this case, the question could be raised whether or not the child's reaction to his mother's wish to marry represented the reaction of "a cheated lover." Was Dean's reaction so devastating because he could not give up his "oedipal victory" and because Mr. Hillard's presence activated his murderous feelings toward his rival? In that case, the therapeutic work would have had to focus on helping the child "accept the reality" that he was replaced by a bigger and more successful rival rather than on the disruption that had occurred in the self-selfobject unit between mother and son with Mr. Hillard's arrival on the scene.

Since the therapist had a self-psychological perspective, the aim of her treatment was the reestablishment of the connection between mother and son. Pathological as this connection was, it was the one that assured the child's self-cohesion. It was hoped that the connection between mother and child would not have to be a pathological one. As long as the mother experienced the child's behavior as defiance, the child continued to feel threatened in his very survival. It was the therapist's empathic response to the mother's own mental state and the fairly consistent interpretation of her own sense of deprivation and need for the child's responsiveness to her that enabled the mother to be empathically accepting of the child. The mother's understanding of Dean's reasons for behaving the way he did provided the selfobject matrix that sufficiently firmed up the child's self to experience the jealousy, rivalry, and possessiveness that had previously overwhelmed him.

We are not stating here that Dean, on his return home, entered the oedipal phase of development, but that the mother's understanding and acceptance of the child's feelings made it more likely that he would be able to experience these affects without becoming overwhelmed by them. Most importantly, it appeared that Dean's relationship with Mr. Hillard promoted a disengagement from his pathological enmeshment with his mother. Thus, Dean had a chance to resume his self-development, in which oedipal experiences might play a more fundamental part in the process of recovery. In addition, Dean now had an opportunity to experience Mr. Hillard as an idealizable male, which was a necessary aspect for the development of his own masculine self.

Our clinical examples have demonstrated the expectable impact of failures in parental empathy on the child at different developmental phases in the child's life. However, there are clinical situations in which it is the parent who becomes symptomatic in response to the changes in the self-selfobject unit in which the child was serving selfobject functions for the parent. The model of the self-selfobject unit is particularly useful in understanding that period in the parents' lives when they more overtly display their expectations of their children and when these expectations are traumatically frustrated. In the early years of the children's lives, the parents' expectations are not easy to detect since these are mainly unconscious. During latency and even more during adolescence, parental expectations become more conscious and more explicit. With the increasing awareness of their expectations, the frustrations of these expectations also become more obvious to the parties involved. The most frequent symptom in the parent following a traumatic loss of the child's selfobject function is depression of varying severity.

Mrs. Silver

Mrs. Silver was 41 years old when she began treatment for symptoms of depression. For about a year she had felt increasingly more irritable, slept poorly, lost interest in many of her activities, and found herself more and more preoccupied with ordinary aches and pains. She eventually had to be hospitalized. During this period she was intensely preoccupied with her oldest son Danny, who had abruptly left law school and went to work instead. It was in the course of her treatment that Danny's vital selfobject function for the mother was recognized.

The mother herself was a promising student but had dropped out of college to marry Danny's father. During her pregnancy she continued her studies but was unable to finish college; she retained a sense of inferiority about herself in having failed to fulfill her scholarly ambitions. She was not conscious of her expectations that Danny, the oldest and the brightest of her children, would complete her own self-development in this respect. This became clear only when she developed a severe depression following the abandonment of his studies. After her recovery from her depression, Mrs. Silver again returned to college and worked very hard to prove to herself that she could excel academically. After she had done very well she gave up college and began to look for other avenues through which she could live up to the ideals of her nuclear self.[5]

Treatment implications

The elucidation of the major acute precipitant to Mrs. Silver's depression led us to focus on the loss of her son's intellectual-professional aspirations. On the surface, this might appear to be offering a very narrow set of explanations for Mrs. Silver's depression, thus, perhaps, simplifying a much more complex web of causative factors. Certainly, her own adverse life experiences and the dynamics of her nuclear family, as well as those of her current family, were multilayered and have undoubtedly codetermined the ensuing depression. However, the treatment process was able to uncover that, for Mrs. Silver, her son represented the embodiment of the intellectual-professional ideals and aspirations of her own nuclear self – ambitions and ideals she had given up at the time of her marriage. This left her with a vulnerability related to this structural deficit in her self. Thus, she essentially failed in the pursuit and fulfillment of her own ambitions and idealized strivings and attached them to her selfobject-son, who was to pursue and attain their fulfillment for her. When her son abruptly turned back on these pursuits, she developed a depressive reaction that was based on this specific core psychopathology. When she another major effort at turning again to these earlier abandoned intellectual pursuits, these were only partially successful because they were to repair the enfeebled and fragmentation-prone self rather than to express its consolidated ambitions and ideals.

It should be noted that whatever complex set of dynamics might be formulated to have originally caused or brought about Mrs. Silver's depression, in the subsequent period of her psychotherapy, the importance of her son as a selfobject was understood and interpreted. It was the specificity of these interpretations that had resulted in the considerable improvement of her depression.

Aging parents and their children

We shall now briefly comment on the aging parent and indicate the usefulness of the model of the self-selfobject unit in this period of the life cycle. This is a period in life when the roles between parent and child are expected to be reversed; a time when it is the parent's self that is placed the center of the unit and the grown child is expected to be empathically encompassing and be responsive to the self-state of the aging parent. However, more often than not, grown children encounter considerable difficulties in experiencing empathy toward their aging parents; the relationship instead is frequently characterized by anger, guilt, and shame. If the now grown children have experienced their parents as having frustrated their own (narcissistic) developmental needs in the past, they are not able to respond to their aging parents empathically. The parents' normally or excessively weakened physical and mental states make them ready targets for their grown children's unconscious need to revenge themselves for past hurts by becoming withholding and unresponsive to them. Since the parents, in many instances, are unaware of having failed their children in any way, they are at a loss to understand children's neglectful, and at times, cruel behavior toward them. Nor are the grown children fully conscious of the source of their need for revenge, since the parents may well have been, in reality, good providers and conscientious in the physical care of their children.

But it is not only aging parents who may suffer from their children's unrelenting need for revenge. The narcissistic rage and the guilt associated with it is a psychological burden for the children as well. Fantasies of telling the parent off and of recounting their childhood hurts are efforts to lighten this burden and to justify their angry withdrawal from their aging parents. The fantasies also express the hope that the parents would accept the responsibility for their anger and by so doing, they would finally demonstrate a capacity for empathy.

Mrs. Kemper

Mrs. Kemper was 62 years old when she consulted with a psychiatrist after having had several years of psychotherapy earlier in her life with another therapist. She was a young-looking woman; her trim and muscular body indicated that she took good care of herself. Indeed, as the therapist learned later, she spent a great deal of time in various sports in which she excelled.

Mrs. Kemper presented her complaints without introduction: Her younger child and only daughter was about to have her first child and the daughter invited her mother-in-law for the postpartum period instead of her own mother. Mrs. Kemper responded to this not only with rage and indignation, but also with considerable concern fearing that this overt rejection by her daughter would result in a complete severance of their relationship. This, she said, would be a repetition of her relationship with her own mother – a circumstance that was her reason for seeking treatment some years before.

Even though Mrs. Kemper came with a problem related to her relationship with her daughter, she began by speaking about her own mother. She gave numerous examples of her mother's emotional unavailability when she was a child and how helpless and childish her mother had become after her parents divorced. As a teenager she took full responsibility for her own, her brother's, and her mother's care and she feared that her mother would pull her back into the same situation now if she did not resist it. The therapist felt that Mrs. Kemper, by focusing on her own childhood, had tried very hard to justify her refusal to visit her now aged and ailing mother. Her repeated statements that she did not feel guilty about this only indicated the considerable guilt she indeed was experiencing.

Mrs. Kemper was married to a rather well-to-do lawyer. Their marriage was a proper but not a particularly intimate relationship. She felt that by bearing two children and bringing them up, she had "repaid" her husband for the emotional and financial independence she had enjoyed in their marriage. She was "a good mother," conscientious in the care of the children; she felt a great deal closer to her son than to her daughter. The daughter grew up to be a serious, studious girl, but rather inhibited in social matters. As the daughter devoted more and more time to her studies and to political and social issues, the mother felt that her daughter considered her frivolous and superficial, and the two women grew farther and farther apart. During the last few years, Mrs. Kemper frequently felt offended by her daughter's "icy attitude" toward her, but the daughter's recent request that the mother not visit her after the baby was born was a particularly heavy blow. She wanted to know what she could do to "repair" this relationship.

The manner in which Mrs. Kemper presented her problem indicated, at first, that she had some insight that there was a connection between her relationship with her mother and that with her daughter. This initial impression, however, was misleading. She continued to be preoccupied with her relationship to her mother and with the need to justify her anger and rejection of her. In relation to the daughter, too, she felt mistreated; she considered herself to have been a good mother and she felt deeply wounded by her daughter's rejection of her.

Treatment implications

What importance does this clinical vignette have for our view of parental dysfunctions? Could we consider this to be an example of generational transmission of faulty parenting? We would regard such an answer to be too general and misleading in the treatment of our patient. The specific features of the mother's parental dysfunction could only have been assessed from the effect that this had on the daughter's development and personality organization. We had no way of assessing that impact. However, we could assess Mrs. Kemper's personality, specifically, how her own childhood experiences had limited her capacity for parental empathy. This would provide us with the understanding of the particular features of her parental dysfunctions and make our interpretations regarding these dysfunctions more specific.

In the course of Mrs. Kemper's treatment, it became clear that it was her mother's "helplessness," her emotional dependency on Mrs. Kemper, that had constituted the childhood (strain) trauma that most powerfully shaped Mrs. Kemper's adult personality. She was a precocious child and her emotional survival depended on her pseudomaturity; she valued most highly her decisiveness and emotional independence. While behaviorally this resulted in a haughty attitude, she remained an emotionally hungry little girl, particularly vulnerable to the rejection by her own children.

It was well into the second year of her treatment that Mrs. Kemper first fully understood her daughter's reason for not inviting her for the postpartum period. The daughter, she had eventually realized, needed someone with her at this time in her life who could be with her without reservations and considerations of her own needs. Mrs. Kemper had to recognize that this was not her daughter's experience with her. The daughter, by not inviting her, was protecting herself from psychic pain, which was no different from Mrs. Kemper's own efforts to protect herself when she refused to visit with her own mother. Only when she had meaningfully linked her daughter's behavior to her own childhood experiences was she able "to forgive" her mother for having failed her as a child.

Acceptance of the limitations of the parents' empathy is a capacity of the adult psyche; not to express revenge against the parents for not having been able to place the child into the center of their universe because of their own narcissistic needs is a developmental accomplishment. Mrs. Kemper was determined to achieve this in her current treatment. As her visits to her mother began to increase and she began to feel better about these, her mother suffered a stroke and had to be placed in a nursing home. In this setting she could accept her mother's helplessness, clingy, and whiny behavior. When, on one of her visits, she was actually able to embrace her mother, which she could not do before, she experienced a peculiar elation and felt that she had indeed accomplished what she wanted in her treatment.

5.6 Conceptual advances in the study of parenting: a summation

To conclude, we shall summarize the essential propositions in this chapter by highlighting the conceptual advances that have already been made on parenting, as well as those that are most likely to follow. This task calls for some broad brush strokes with which to place parenting as a developmental achievement firmly within the whole of self-development.

The nature versus nurture controversy regarding the development of the self in health and illness has also encompassed the functions and capacities of parenting. Benedek, the most widely recognized psychoanalyst who worked in this area, postulated a biological readiness for motherliness through hormonal regulation that evolves out of the experiences of pregnancy and lactation. However, while the initial impetus for mothering in the postpartum period is a hormonally determined potentiality, mothering beyond infancy could not be explained on a hormonal or biological basis, nor could the increasingly more significant functions of fathering. Parenting beyond the early phases requires the recognition of psychological mechanisms. Regarding these, Benedek [8] elaborated on the process of identification in the following way. The mother, as a caretaker, identifies with her own mother and, at the same time, she identifies with her infant's receptive needs by regressively reexperiencing her own infancy.

Benedek's theory of motherliness, evolving out of a physiological (i.e., hormonal) regulation, has found general acceptance in psychoanalysis. Her explanation as to what sustains motherliness throughout the child's development, however, has to be questioned. The assumption that identification would create fixed, unchangeable patterns of parenting was not in keeping with clinical observations. Clinical observations indicate that parenting usually undergoes necessary changes in relation to the same child and in relation to the various children of the same parents. The theory of identification also could not account for the structural changes that take place in the adult self in relation to parenting as Benedek had postulated. It is because of these structural changes that she had maintained that parenthood was a genuine developmental phase.

In this chapter, we have suggested that: (1) the observation that parental behavior is flexible (e.g., it changes in relation to the same child in terms of the child's increasingly complex and constantly changing psychic organization as well as in relation to the varied temperaments and inborn capacities of various children) can best be explained with the adults' capacity for attunement with the child (i.e., with parental empathy); and (2) the structural changes in the adult in relation to parenting are intimately related to the narcissistic (selfobject) nature of the parentchild tie.

The developmental significance of parental empathy has been confirmed by current infant research, in which it has been repeatedly demonstrated that the infant, born with "a genetic ground plan" has to be assured of phase-appropriate environmental responses if this groundplan is to develop into a viable, vigorous, and creative human psyche. These specific phase-appropriate environmental responses are the ones that self psychology calls "selfobject functions."

Our conceptualization of parenting is based on Kohut's self psychology, which recognizes the central importance of empathy as a mode of observation as well as an emotional nutrient and its failures in parenting to be of major pathogenic significance. In relation to empathy as a mode of observation, we have emphasized that parental empathy requires not only a temporary immersion into the inner world of the child, but a sustained capacity to perceive the child's affects and his particular manner of protecting himself from the potentially destructive (i.e., overstimulating) impact of his emotional environment. This capacity for adult empathy (i.e., when the parent, after having briefly experienced the child's affects, maintains his sense of separateness) is the hallmark of successful transformation of infantile narcissism into its adult form. The capacity for empathy is, therefore, a reliable indicator of the completion of adult self-development, which also includes the capacity for the regulation of tension, affect, and self-esteem, along with the development of other mature psychic functions such as wisdom, humor, and the ability to contemplate one's own transience. By placing the capacity for empathy into the center of parental functions, we have linked parenting inextricably to self-development.

When we consider that parental functions cannot be grafted onto the parents' personalities since these are functions of the parents' own nuclear self, we can appreciate that successful parenting depends on the parental selves being fully consolidated, that they had "formed stable patterns of ambitions and ideals," and that "the parental selves are experiencing the unrolling of the expression of these patterns along a finite life curve that leads from a preparative beginning through an active, productive, creative middle to a fulfilled end" [28].

> It makes no difference at which point of the life curve the parental selves are during the oedipal phase of the child; so long as the pattern of the parental self is clearly designed and well consolidated and is in the process of expressing itself, the fulfilling peak and the fulfilled end are already implied. The oedipal child then is the beneficiary of the fact that the parents are in narcissistic balance. If the little boy feels that his father looks on him proudly as a "chip off the old block" and allows him to merge with him and with his adult greatness, then his oedipal phase will be a decisive step in self-consolidation and self-pattern firming, including the laying down of one of the several variants of integrated maleness – despite the unavoidable frustrations of his sexual and competitive aspirations and despite the unavoidable conflicts caused by ambivalence and mutilation fears.
>
> (p. 234)

In the course of development, parental empathy will expectedly fluctuate since it is subject to ordinary life stresses.[6] However, such ordinary fluctuations in parental empathy are nontraumatic since they are part of a progressive developmental process. Only failures in parental empathy that are sustained over long periods of time indicate a defect in the parent's own self-development.

The close linkage between parenting and self-development is further justified by the narcissistic nature of the parent-child tie. The narcissistic nature of parental love assures parental care but it is also this quality of the relationship that makes parenting a particularly vulnerable adult function. In self psychology the narcissistic nature of the parent-child tie is encompassed by the concept of the selfobject. It is this concept that permits a fresh approach to the study of parenting by bringing together experientially and conceptually what the extrospective observer could only regard as "internal" or "external" in relation to development and pathogenesis. Since the parent as a selfobject is always viewed from the vantage point of the experiencing self of the infant or child, the external environment may thus be consistently studied as part of the inner world of the particular child.

The significance of selfobject functions extends throughout development and is not restricted to the early years of the child's life. The transformation of infantile grandiosity and exhibitionism into vigor, vitality, and self-esteem (through phase-appropriate mirroring) and the establishment of valued ideals (through repeated merger experiences with the idealized values of the selfobjects) is not completed during the first few years of life; self-assertive, grandiose, and exhibitionistic needs are in evidence throughout childhood, and ideals and goals of the nuclear self become firmed up only during adolescence. Though the extent and nature of these selfobject functions change with increasing differentiation and structuralization of the child's psyche, with physical growth, with the acquisition of new skills and, with the tentative expression of innate talents, the child's growing self continually needs to be validated by affirmative selfobject responses. This indicates that the psyche is more appropriately viewed as an open system, retaining its capacity for structural change, though to a progressively lesser degree, over the whole of the life cycle. It is this lifelong need for empathic selfobject responsiveness that best explains the parents' own needs to be affirmed by their children in their parenting capacity. Nothing assures such affirmation better than the child's wholesome and progressive development and, conversely, nothing can "erode" the parents' empathic capacity as quickly as a child who becomes symptomatic. We have suggested that this inherent reciprocity in the relationship is most aptly expressed in the model of the self-selfobject unit. This model is useful because the clinician can either focus on the child's self and examine it in relation to the parental selfobject or he or she can focus on the parent's self in order to examine the nature of parental dysfunctions and determine the manner in which the child is being used as the parent's selfobject.

Using the self-selfobject model, we can appreciate that it is not the overt psychopathology of the parent (which is visible to the external observer and in response to which the child may find various modes of coping), but it is the more subtle, invisible deficiency or absence of certain key functions that will have pathogenic influence. The impact, for instance, of the absence of the gleam in the mother's eyes or the lack of firmness in her arms when she holds her baby can only be discovered from within the experience of the child (or, reconstructively, in the treatment of an adult patient).

It should now be evident that both "identification" and "adaptation," especially with a frustrating caretaker, are not only phenomena noted by the external observer in relation to the social interaction between parent and child, but that these are already the results of a troubled and troubling inter-action. Thus, the infant's or child's identification with the aggressor impinges on self-development and necessitates the variety of compromises in relation to the potentials of the developing self. These compromises have been described as "the false self" [49], "defensive structures" [28], and assuring "adaptations" to an "average nonexpectable environment" [24]. In all instances, they serve as a shield to protect the "true self" [49] or the "nuclear self" [27].

Our clinical examples indicate only a very small fraction of the infinite variety of situations in which the model of the self-selfobject unit aids the clinician in the diagnosis and treatment of parental dysfunctions. In discussing the cases of three young children, we hoped to indicate that the interference with parental empathy may be related to various levels of self-pathology in the parent. For example, Martin's mother had hoped to make child rearing into her "career" and thereby buttress her diminishing self-esteem, while Bobby's mother used her son as a selfobject in a more fundamental way – to protect her fragile self from fragmentation.

We have demonstrated our approach to treatment with the case of Dean. In addition to the therapeutic efforts in this case, we have illustrated that a child whose self has not attained adequate consolidation is not able to experi-ence the passions traditionally associated with the Oedipus complex, namely, rivalry, jealousy, and possessiveness, without untoward effects. We also want to emphasize that even when the child has attained adequate consolidation of the self and could experience these affects without adverse consequences, the child is still in need of the affirmative responsiveness of the parents in relation to these affects. In other words, it is not only parental seductiveness, counter-aggression, or counter-rivalry that may create the pathogenic conditions: the very absence of affirmative acceptance of a child's rivalry and possessiveness directed at the parents is of pathogenic significance.

In connection with Mrs. Kemper, we could raise the question regarding the role identification plays in the transmission of the dysfunction of parent-ing. It could be argued that Mrs. Kemper's parental dysfunction was related to her identification with her own mother. However, we would maintain that such an interpretation would neither describe the process of transmission nor would it be useful in the treatment process since it would fail to take into consideration Mrs. Kemper's personality organization and the manner in which this had determined the nature of her specific parental dysfunctions. In fact, identification with the parent's own parents is an inadequate explanation of the "generational transmission" of parental dysfunctions because, when we see such transmissions in clinical practice, the nature and extent of parental dysfunctions are not identical in the two generations. In the case of Mrs. Kemper, for example, in order to diagnose the specific features of her parental dysfunctions, we had to link these to the specific features of her self-disorder; this disorder in Mrs. Kemper found a very different expression than in her mother. Mrs. Kemper's mother was a helpless woman who, unable to respond to her daughter's needs, had expected and received considerable support from her (i.e., Mrs. Kemper was a parenting child). As an adult, in order to protect herself from further traumatization, she developed a haughty, pseudoindependence as a defense. Though proper in her behavior as a mother, she remained centered on her own needs. This created a parental dysfunction very different from her own mother's: Rather than "burdening" her daughter with her selfobject needs, she remained aloof and self-centered. When the daughter did not invite Mrs. Kemper to share one of her most important life experiences with her, she (the daughter) protected herself from the hurt of her mother's aloofness and, at the same time, she expressed her rage at the mother for not having been emotionally available to her during her childhood. Since Mrs. Kemper sought help specifically related to her parental dysfunction, treatment could focus on this rather exclusively. However, whether or not she will be successful in building a new relationship with her daughter will depend on the daughter's willingness to "forgive" her mother in the manner in which Mrs. Kemper was eventually able to forgive her own mother.

Notes

1 The concepts of "selfobject" and "selfobject functions" will be elaborated upon later. At this time, we only want to stress that selfobject functions (e.g., the mirroring and merger with an idealized adult) are silent but active adult functions, and that the building up of psychological structures is conceptualized here as occurring through the transmuting internalization of these functions. This theory of structure formation has to be differentiated from one in which it is hypothesized that structure formation occurs through the internalization of good and bad objects.

2 For more information, see reference 5.

3 What we are stating here is a considerable modification of an earlier formulation by Ornstein [38a] regarding the relationship between adaptation and the concept of the selfobject: "... the concept of the selfobject serves as a bridge across which intrapsychic, developmental-genetic determinants of health and illness can be integrated with the psychosocial determinants. The new integration also permits the notion of mere adjustment to external reality to be clearly differentiated from a metapsychologically sophisticated conception of *adaptation* to reality."

4 The distinction between primary, compensatory, and defensive psychic structures is a useful one [28]. Primary structures develop in relation to optimal, phase-appropriate

responses to narcissistic developmental needs. These are the structures that are responsible for the healthy functioning of the self, for the consolidation of both poles (ambitions and ideals), and the full utilization of innate skills and talents; the self is experienced as cohesive and vigorous. But if the developmental unfolding of the grandiose self meets with traumatic dysfunction of empathy on the part of the primary selfobject, the resulting defects in the self will be covered over with defensive structure that will prevent further unfolding and structuralization of the pole of the ambitions. However, if the child has an opportunity to turn to other available selfobjects, this will ensure the building up of psychic structure at either of the two poles and lead to the development of compensatory structures. If well consolidated, these structures will afford the self-sufficient functional freedom, safeguard its cohesiveness, and allow the progression of further development.

5 Kohut [28] speaks of the early development of a core self – the "nuclear self." "This structure is the basis for our sense of being an independent center of initiative and perception, integrated with our most central ambitions and ideals and our experience that our body and mind form a unit in space and continuum in time. This cohesive and enduring psychic configuration, in connection with a correlated set of talents and skills that it attracts to itself or that develops in response to the demands of the ambitions and ideals of the nuclear self form the central sector of the personality. The nuclear self (a bipolar structure) has three major constituents: the grandiose-exhibitionistic self at one pole and the idealized parent image at the other, with innate skills and talents between them. Once the nuclear self is established and after ... having become independent of the genetic factors that determined its specific shape and content, strives only ... to live out its intrinsic potentialities." These intrinsic potentialities, the "ground plan" or "life program" of the nuclear self, are central motivating structures within the bipolar self.

6 In a small but well conceived study, Letourneau has demonstrated that, contrary to general belief, life stresses do not affect parental empathy [31].

References

1 Abelin, E. Some further observations and comments on the earliest role of the father. *Int. J. Psychoanal.* 56: 293, 1975.

2 Ainsworth, M. The Development of Infant-Mother Attachment. In B. Caldwell and R. Ricciuti (Eds.), *Review of Child Developmental Research*, Vol. 3. Chicago: University of Chicago Press, 1973. Pp. 1–94.

3 Anthony, E. J. A clinical evaluation of children with psychotic parents. *Am. J. Psychiatry* 126: 177, 1969.

4 Anthony, E. J. The family and the psychoanalytic process in children. *Psychoanal. Study Child* 35: 3, 1980.

5 Atwood, G. E., and Stolorow, R. D. *Structures of Subjectivity: Explorations in Psychoanalytic Psychotherapy.* Hillsdale, New Jersey: Analytic Press, 1984.

6 Barnett, R. K., Hofer, L., and Stern, D. *Dyadic Interactive Process Profile (DIPP): A Measure of Social Interactive Behaviors and Style.* Presented to the Third International Conference on Infant Studies, Austin, Texas, March, 1982 (unpublished manuscript).

7 Basch, M. F. The concept of affect: A re-examination. *J. Am. Psychoanal. Assoc.* 24: 759, 1976.

8 Benedek, T. Toward the biology of the depressive constellation. *J. Am. Psychoanal. Assoc.* 4: 389, 1956.

9 Benedek, T. Parenthood as a developmental phase. *J. Am. Psychoanal. Assoc.* 7: 380, 1959.

10 Benedek, T. Motherhood and Nurturing. In E. J. Anthony and T. Benedek (Eds.), *Parenthood: Its Psychology and Psychopathology*. Boston: Little, Brown, 1970.

11 Benedek, T. Parenthood During the Life Cycle. In E. J. Anthony and T. Benedek (Eds.), *Parenthood: Its Psychology and Psychopathology*. Boston: Little, Brown, 1970.

12 Benedek, T. The Psychobiology of Pregnancy. In E. J. Anthony and T. Benedek (Eds.), *Parenthood: Its Psychology and Psychopathology*. Boston: Little, Brown, 1970.

13 Bowlby, J. *Attachment and Loss*, Vol. 1. New York: Basic Books, 1969.

14 Brody, S. Continuity and Conflict in Maternal Behavior. Panel on: "Parenthood as a Developmental Phase" reported by H. Parens. *J. Am. Psychoanal. Assoc.* 23: 154, 1975.

15 Brody, S. The concepts of attachment and bonding. Paper delivered at the First International Congress on Infant Psychiatry, Estoril, Portugal, May 1980.

16 Burlingham, D. T., Goldberger, A., and Lussier, A. Simultaneous analysis of mother and child. *Psychoanal. Study Child* 10: 165, 1955.

17 Chess, S., and Thomas, A. Infant bonding: Mystique and reality. *Am. J. Orthopsychiatry* 52(2): 213, 1982.

18 Demos, V. Empathy and Affect, Reflections on Infant Experience. In J. Lichtenberg, M. Bornstein, and D. Silver (Eds.), *Empathy II*. Hillsdale, New Jersey: Analytic Press, 1984.

19 Erikson, E. On the generational cycle: An address. *Int. J. Psychoanal.* 61: 213, 1980.

20 Fliess, R. The metapsychology of the analyst. *Psychoanal. Q.* 11: 211, 1942.

21 Freud, S. On narcissism: An introduction (1914). In J. Strachey (Ed.), *The Standard Edition of the Complete Psychological Works of Sigmund Freud*. London: Hogarth, 1957. Vol. 14, Pp. 67–102.

22 Freud, S. Introductory lectures on psychoanalysis (1916/17). *Standard Edition*. 1963. Vol. 16.

23 Greenspan, S. I. *Psychopathology and Adaptation in Infancy and Early Childhood: Principles of Clinical Diagnosis and Preventive Intervention*. Clinical Infant Reports Series of the National Center for Clinical Infant Programs. No. 1, 1981.

24 Hartmann, H. *Ego Psychology and the Problem of Adaptation*. New York: International Universities Press, 1958.

25 Herzog, J. M. On Father Hunger: The Father's Role in the Modulation of Aggressive Drive and Fantasy. In S. H. Cath, A. Gurwitt, and J. M. Ross (Eds.), *Father and Child: Developmental and Clinical Perspectives*. Boston: Little, Brown, 1982.

26 Klaus, M., and Kennell, J. H. Human maternal behavior at the first contact with the young. *Pediatrics* 46: 187, 1976.

27 Kohut, H. *The Analysis of the Self*. New York: International Universities Press, 1971.

28 Kohut, H. *The Restoration of the Self*. New York: International Universities Press, 1977.

29 Kohut, H. The two analyses of Mr. Z. *Int. J. Psychoanal.* 60: 3, 1979.

30 Lax, R. F. Some aspects of the interaction between mother and impaired child: Mother's narcissistic trauma. *Int. J. Psychoanal.* 53: 339, 1972.

31 Letourneau, C. Empathy and stress: How they affect parental aggression. *Soc. Work* 26: 383, 1981.

32 Lichtenberg, J. Reflections on the first year of life. *Psychoanalytic Inquiry* 1: 695, 1982.

33 Lozoff, B., Brittenham, G. M., and Trause, M. A. The mother-newborn relationship: Limits of adaptability. *J. Pediatr.* 91: 1, 1977.

34 Mahler, M. S. Thoughts about development and individuation. *Psychoanal. Study Child* 18: 307, 1963.

35 Mahler, M. S., Pine, F., and Bergman, A. *The Psychological Birth of the Human Infant.* New York: Basic Books, 1975.

36 Olden, C. On adult empathy with children. *Psychoanal. Study Child* 8: 111, 1953.

37 Ornstein, A. Self-pathology in childhood: Developmental and clinical considerations. *Psychiatr. Clin. North Am.* 4: 435, 1981.

38 Ornstein, A. An Idealizing Transference of the Oedipal Phase. In J. D. Lichenberg, and S. Kaplan (Eds.), *Reflections on Self Psychology.* Hillsdale, N.J.: Analytic Press, 1983. pp. 135–148.

38a Ornstein, P. H. Self Psychology and the Concept of Health. In A. Goldberg (Ed.), *Advances in Self Psychology.* New York: International Universities Press, 1980.

39 Parens, H. Panel on "Parenthood as a Developmental Phase." *J. Am. Psychoanal. Assoc.* 23: 154, 1975.

40 Paul, N. L. Parental Empathy. In E. J. Anthony and T. Benedek (Eds.), *Parenthood: Its Psychology and Psychopathology.* Boston: Little, Brown, 1970.

41 Rutter, M. *Maternal Deprivation Reassessed.* Middlesex, England: Penguin Books, 1972.

42 Sander, L. Issues in early mother-child interaction. *J. Am. Acad. Child Psychiatry* 1: 141, 1962.

43 Sander, L. Infant and Caretaking Environment: Investigation and Conceptualization of Adaptive Behavior in a System of Increasing Complexity. In E. J. Anthony (Ed.), *Exploration in Child Psychiatry.* New York: Plenum, 1975.

44 Schafer, R. Generative empathy in the treatment situation. *Psychoanal. Q.* 28: 347, 1959.

45 Steele, B. F. Parental Abuse of infants and Small Children. In E. J. Anthony and T. Benedek (Eds.), *Parenthood: Its Psychology and Psychopathology.* Boston: Little, Brown, 1970.

46 Stern, D. *The First Relationship: Infant and Mother.* Cambridge, Mass: Harvard University Press, 1977.

47 Tolpin, M. On the beginnings of a cohesive self: An application of the concept of transmuting internalization to the study of transitional object and signal anxiety. *Psychoanal. Study Child* 26: 316, 1971.

48 Tolpin, M., and Kohut, H. The Disorders of the Self: The Psychopathology of the First Years of Life. In S. I. Greenspan and G. H. Pollock (Eds.), *The Course of Life. Psychoanalytic Contributions Toward Understanding Personality Development, Vol. I, Infancy and Early Childhood,* NIMH, 1980.

49 Winnicott, D. W. *Maturational Processes and the Facilitating Environment: Studies in the Theory of Emotional Development.* New York: International Universities Press, 1965.

50 Winnicott, D. W. *Playing and Reality.* New York: Basic Books, 1971.

6 Anne and Vivienne
The early adolescence of two young teenagers

Anna Ornstein

In their book *Early Adolescence and the Search for the Self: A Developmental Perspective*, Douglas and Barbara Schave delineate early adolescence from latency and the later phases of adolescence by pointing to the distinct characteristics of this age group's cognitive, emotional and social development. The theory that had informed their clinical observations and served as the organizer of their theoretical position was psychoanalytic self psychology: the development of the self, as this is conceptualized to occur in an empathically-responsive selfobject environment.

In order to elucidate the psychological make-up of the early adolescent, the Schaves make careful comparisons between the psychological tasks of toddlerhood and early adolescence. Their thorough review of the literature tends to obscure the essential features of the developmental period that is the major concern of the book and creates unnecessary repetitions in the text.

6.1 The "softening" of psychic structures during the toddler years and during early adolescence

In contrast to traditional developmental theory, the Schaves do not consider puberty and the attendant physical changes to be responsible for the psychological changes that usher in adolescence. Rather, they consider the changes in cognition, the change from concrete to operational thinking, to be the primary organizer of this forward move in development.

In their view, in toddlerhood and in early adolescence, far-reaching psychological changes are ushered in by a "quantum leap" in cognition. In the toddler years, the leap is made from sensorimotor to preoperational, and in pre-adolescence, from concrete to formal operational thinking. In both instances, the changes that are thereby introduced "soften" the psychic structures, which, potentially, allow a higher level of psychological organization.

However, such softening also renders the psyche particularly vulnerable and "egocentric." In both developmental periods, dialectics are set up between striving for autonomy and emotional independence on the one hand, and an increased need for attachment and validation by the environment on the other. The need for autonomy and independence constitute a challenge to the environment and may make acceptance and empathic responsiveness of the toddler's and early adolescent's behavior extremely difficult. In other words, just as the need for acceptance and validation increases, empathic failures on the part of the environment are most likely to occur. How well these development periods will be negotiated will depend on the environment's capacity to be responsive to the child's internal struggle, rather than respond punitively to the changed behavior, behavior that may bewilder parents and make demands on them that they may not be able to meet because of the limitation of their own emotional resources.

It is the failure on the part of the child's emotional environment to appreciate the nature of the child's internal struggle to maintain psychological equilibrium that accounts for the presence of what the authors call "primitive defenses," such as disavowal and denial. Here, as in all other periods of development, defenses serve the crucial function of maintaining self-cohesion. In other words, such "primitive defenses" become necessary when the toddler's and child's increased vulnerability is not being responded to with acceptance and understanding. These defense operations constitute the building blocks for the development of psychopathology later in life.

6.2 The relationship between the developmental tasks of toddlerhood and early adolescence

The authors discuss in great detail the similarities and differences between the developmental tasks of the toddler years and early adolescence, but the significance of the relationship between the two, and what particular developmental aspects of the toddler years will become clinically decisive for the early adolescent is not clearly stated. What will prove to be clinically decisive for early adolescence as well as for all later periods of development, is the cohesion of the self, whether or not the young child has been able to establish a relatively cohesive self without development-crippling needs for defensive operations. A self that is vigorous and had developed the capacity to regulate anxiety and various kinds of affects will be able to negotiate the psychological changes as these occur in early adolescence: the "cognitive leap" and the increase in sexuality, the latter an inevitable consequence of puberty.

While the primary developmental task of the first few years of life is the establishment of self-cohesion, the primary developmental task of adolescence is the establishment of relatively firm ideals. Both these developmental accomplishments have a decisive impact on the young teen's capacity to develop a reliable and relatively independent self-esteem regulatory system. Difficulty in maintaining a relatively stable self-esteem indicates that the strains of early adolescence have overtaxed the child's psyche. If the self had remained fragmentation- and/or depletion-prone, if it had to resort to the excessive use of denial and disavowal and other forms of defensive operations, this will limit its capacity to reach a higher level of organization in response to the "softening" of its psychic structures.

Defects in self-development do not become manifest until the time when the psyche is called upon to master developmental challenges for which it was inadequately prepared. The challenges in the cognitive and somatic realms of early adolescence place a special demand on the cohesiveness of the self: it is the early adolescent who can articulate the sense of ·inner emptiness or a "black whole" but it was the unmirrored toddler who had originally experienced it.

6.3　The selfobject needs of the toddler and the early adolescent

However – and this is crucial in our consideration – "the softening" of the psychic structures during early adolescence also provides a new opportunity to compensate for the deficits that earlier periods in life may have left behind. This requires that the child's emotional environment recognize these new opportunities. Such an opportunity was presented to Vivienne[1] by her teacher, John May.

Vivienne Loomis was a ninth grade student when she committed suicide. She was 14 years and 4 months old at the time. In the sixth grade, Vivienne developed "a crush," an intense idealization on her teacher, John May. John knew that he was important to Vivienne but only after the suicide did he know how important he was – or maybe not even then. "I believe I will lose my life because you are not here," writes Vivienne to John after he left the school. "You see there have been a lot of tears lately. Not where anyone would see, but just by myself. I think I am lonely or something related to it. But there is nobody who can help me. I was just wondering if you would please send me something encouraging, positive, anything! for me to live on. It's funny but I have really gone to pieces ..." (p. 49).

It is not difficult to understand Vivienne's feelings for John. John, a young enthusiastic teacher, spotted Vivienne and another girl who had been outcasts in their sixth grade class. He wanted to improve these girls' self-esteem, to increase their self-confidence. He recognized and deeply appreciated Vivienne as a specially gifted and sensitive child; he read her poetry carefully and responded to it with admiration and helpful suggestions. He also told her that she was beautiful as Vivienne was convinced that she was not. John could not have known how deeply this might effect an extremely vulnerable early adolescent. When John left, Vivienne did not only suffer the loss of John himself. More importantly, what she lost were the *feelings* she had experienced when John focused on her exclusively and when he, without reservations, accepted her as she was. John May was a teacher and a friend and not a therapist, he could not have been aware of the depth of Vivienne's needs and that such deeply felt needs to be reassured cannot be undone by praise and reassurance. Most importantly, John could not have known that once provided, Vivienne's self was too fragile to tolerate the absence of his understanding and genuine caring. The time they had together was not sufficient for the internalization of the selfobject functions which, at this time in Vivienne's life, only he could provide.

I agree with Mack's interpretations of John May's importance to Vivienne. He says that the task of finding serviceable ideals with which adolescents must struggle, was here loaded with the additional burden of repairing an injured self and redeeming the crippled sense of Vivienne's own worth. I shall quote Mack: "… the loss of love objects such as John May, who has been idealized in order to fulfill redemptive or reparative needs, becomes a precipitant of suicide *by virtue of the essential function the person serves in maintaining the very structure of the self*" (p. 184, italics mine).

The significance of idealization during this developmental period can be seen in the adolescent's persistent and pervasive need to be merged with the idealized other. The need appears to be ubiquitous. The idealization of charismatic leaders, rock stars, movie idols, and peers, sustain many a young adolescent during this potentially turbulent period in their lives.

When comparing the toddler years and adolescence, it has to be emphasized that the selfobject functions that the environment has to provide are not identical in the two developmental periods. The toddler's need for mirroring, the enthusiastic responsiveness that is essential for the toddler's ability to experience exhilaration that accompanies the performance of rapidly-acquired new skills, shifts in early adolescence to the need to be merged with an idealized other. In contrast to the archaic merger experiences of the infant, in which the infant and the young child are merged with the parents physical power, in early adolescence, the capacity for formal operational thinking enables adolescents to long for attributes of personality they feel they do not possess. In addition to people, they are now also capable of appreciating abstract ideas and to put these on a pedestal. This is the age for intense and passionate idealization of either people or ideas, or both. The passion, the very intensity of the longing to become part of a person with highly valued attributes or universal ideals (political or religious), makes the early adolescent particularly vulnerable to disillusionments. Not being able to merge with an idealized other, or ideals as these may be represented by a single person, (such as a guru) or their own peer group, has a profound effect on the early adolescent's self-esteem. Feeling dejected and emotionally isolated creates a traumatic drop in an already precarious self-esteem system, that may result in suicidal ideations, suicide attempts, and, not too infrequently, in successfully completed suicides.

Not that mirroring and validation are no longer necessary. Rather, that mirroring had now become more specific: it is longed for from the particular other or others who are idealized. It is now that young teenagers may become obsessed with their value to others; comparing themselves to others can leave them feeling wanting in qualities such as courage, intelligence, strength, or beauty. Feeling merged with others who embody these attributes, or represent valued ideals, provide the enfeebled self, at least temporarily, with a sense of power and worthwhileness.

Vivienne's diary documents her preoccupation with such ideals from the time she was 11½ years old. She was uncompromising in her quest. She wanted "perfect sensitivity, understanding, generosity, friendliness, kindness, compassion ..." John May fulfilled these expectations. He was the only one she could look up to, who met her demand for perfection: she could idealize him, and he in turn, was optimally "mirroring" her. The hope that Vivienne placed in John as a potential redeemer of her enfeebled self was traumatically destroyed when he failed to respond to her pleading for reassurance. It was then that she experienced herself without any value, a burden to others and it was then that she began to contemplate suicide.

6.4 Aggression, sexuality, and the cohesion of the self

I believe the authors of this book minimize the importance of the impact that the pubertal child's emerging sexuality has on development. Sexual "energies" now become available that had not been available before. If the toddler years left the psyche fragmentation-prone, sexualization of relationships may become a major avenue through which the pubertal – and later the adolescent and adult – may be able to maintain self-cohesion·and continue to function.

The sexualization of the need to maintain contact with an indifferent or abusive environment has to be distinguished from the joyful experiences of changes in the body of the pubertal child who had entered this period of life with a relatively intact self.

One of the most beautiful descriptions of these experiences can be found in the diary of Anne Frank. (2) Anne's description of her awakening sexuality would indicate that this was a youngster who was, developmentally, well prepared to deal with the physical changes of puberty. The changes in her body opened up a new dimension and further enriched her already rich and creative psychological life. Anne wrote that a girl in the years of puberty becomes quiet within and began to think about the wonders that where happening in her body. She discovered that she had experienced that, too. Anne was thinking that what had been happening to her was so wonderful and not only could have been seen on her body-but all that was taking place inside. Each time she had her period – and that had only been three times – she has had the feeling that in spite of all the pain, unpleasantness and nastiness, she had a sweet secret – and that was why – although it was nothing but a nuisance to her in a way – she always longed for the time that she was feeling that secret within her again (p. 116). In the weeks and months that follow, Anne describes the welling up of sexual feelings. She said that she believed it was spring within her, she felt that spring was awakening. She felt it in her whole body and soul. It was an effort for her to behave normally because she felt utterly confused-she didn't know what to read, what to write, what to do-she only knew that she was longing. (p. 136.). Describing her reactions to Peter's (1) adoring looks, she wrote that he had given her such a gentle and warm look which had made a tender glow within her. She recalled that if he looked at her with those eyes that laughed and winked, then it was as if a little light went on inside of her. (p. 139). It is instructive to compare Anne's experience of her budding sexuality, its· joyfulness, and the way it enhanced her now rapidly expanding self-experiences to Vivienne's. From her sister we learn that Vivienne never felt comfortable about her body and her appearance. She tended toward overweight and after the age of ten, when, because of a rapid growth of her abdomen she had undergone a pelvic examination, her feelings toward sexuality began to range widely. She had no intimate relationships but, at the same time, she had exposed herself to situations where she could have been sexually exploited, and at one time was almost raped. She felt indifferent toward these crude advances and rape attempts, a response that one suspects had to be defensive against their potentially traumatic impact.

The hallmark of a cohesive self that is not compromised by disavowal, denial, and other defensive operations is its capacity to experience strong affects without the threat of fragmentation. This is as true for negative effects as it is for sexual passions. There is no hint in Vivienne's diary and poems that she experienced rage at her mother. Anne Frank, on the other hand, was open in her criticism of her mother; many passages of the diary are taken up with the description of her mother's inadequacies. Repeatedly, Anne returns to her disappointment in her mother, who was no longer the idealized figure of her childhood. How badly she wanted to reinstate such idealization! She says: "I have in my eyes image what a perfect mother and wife should be; and in her whom I must call 'mother,' I find no trace of that image" (p. 41).

Katherine Dalsimer in an article "Female Adolescent Development; A Study of *The Diary of Anne Frank*,"[1] considers this the expression of Anne's Oedipal conflict. She interprets Anne's rages at her mother as "an attempt to free herself from a bond which, with the welling up of adult impulses, is experienced as having homosexual overtones" (p. 500).

Whatever the origin of Anne's feelings toward her mother and whatever functions these may have served in the evolution of her femininity, Anne is experiencing these affects in their full force – and most importantly appears to have no guilt associated with them.

6.5 Anne's and Vivienne's early life experiences

Many of the answers, related to the question as to the origin of the differences between the self-organizations of these two early adolescents, may be found in the difference in their respective psychological organizations prior to this period.

All we know of Anne's early life is what we can infer from her diary. Information about Vivienne's early childhood were obtained from interviews with Vivienne's siblings and parents by Mack and Hickler.

Vivienne was the youngest of three children. The authors characterized Vivienne's family as warm and intelligent with deep moral concerns.

Vivienne's father was a minister, a man of integrity and high moral standards, who was indecisive and self-sacrificing. The mother, a "modern woman," was definite and crisp in her manner of relating but absorbed in her own struggles. The household revolved around the mother's frame of mind, she was ambitious for creative achievement both for herself and her children. She focused on Vivienne in particular as the child appeared artistically precocious.

As an infant, her mother said, Vivienne made very few demands and required much less attention than her two older siblings. However, her siblings remembered that Vivienne had many tantrums, that she would scream for hours at times. "My mother was always sick, always tired ... she needed attention," Vivienne's sister said. "Sometimes she got attention by making people feel guilty. She would make it seem that we were doing things to hurt her" (p. 9).

When Vivienne was 2 years old, her parents went to Europe for 10 weeks. The authors concluded that "... at two Vivienne's response to her mother after the ten week separation seems to reflect the early alienation between them, and by three she pitted herself against her mother with an intense stubbornness. By age 4½, Vivienne had already developed the sensitivity that made her vulnerable to depression and suicide. She showed even then her unusual empathy for the sufferings of others, her ability to identify with their pain. Most compelling was her need to assume her family's griefs and burdens" (p. 93).

Mother made Vivienne her confidante: "She was such a good listener ... I would say to her 'Well what would you do –' and she would give me advice" the mother reported. Vivienne, recognizing this need in her mother, called her "My Little Princess," the one she had a cheer up and keep in narcissistic balance.

What we have here is a "parenting child." A child, who, in order to remain in emotional contact with her mother entered the mother's inner world, who could not enter hers. I believe the special sensitivity that Vivienne developed toward the pain of others was the direct consequence of her need to seek her mother out in this manner. Only once did she complain about this in a letter to John May: "Mommy came to me for help. And I really have helped her whenever I could. But it puts a certain pressure on me; I am not fourteen yet, and Mommy is forty-eight."

Such a relationship between parent and child has tremendous significance for the development of the self, and therefore, for later development. The first and most obvious consequence of this is that the child is deprived of her own developmental need to be in the center of the parent's universe, to be mirrored in her own right. Deprived of the developmentally-needed mirroring selfobject responses, the self remains feeble and fragmentation-prone.

Mother thought of Vivienne as a child who made no demands on her and was content to be by herself, while her siblings remembered the temper tantrums and the long periods of crying. Eventually, a child who is not being responded to will give up demanding attention. This, I believe, is the onset of a childhood depression, a time when a child withdraws into herself and begins to experience the abyss of a black hole, a sense of emptiness where – under optimal circumstances – liveliness and enthusiasm ought to reside. This is the child who develops a certain kind of precocity that successfully hides the defects and deficits in the self that are the legacy of the environment's failure to have heard her cry and respond to her legitimate need be soothed and comforted.

If later in life, the child becomes "special" to someone else, this becomes a new opportunity to achieve self-cohesion belatedly. Had Vivienne been able to internalize John May's unconditional acceptance of her, this could have been such an opportunity. His departure and failure to respond to her pleading, robbed her of any hope to experience herself as a human being who was lovable and deserved to live.

Eventually, Vivienne became fascinated by death as something sacred and true while life was full of disappointments: "I have come to consider death an emotional, deep, and poetical fact of life." Vivienne had successfully transformed death from something dreaded and bleak to an idealized realm. Death became a solution for her by virtue of being considered the perfect and self-completing object she had always been seeking. A most unexpected place to discover the need to be merged with the perfection of another!

In order to explain the suicide, John Mack takes the reader back to the child's earliest experiences. He is careful in pointing out that the disappointment during early adolescence, no matter how severe, is not sufficient to explain the destruction of the self. For Vivienne, "the hurts of this period would not in themselves have been decisive, but they built upon deeper damage to the self that occurred during the earliest years."

6.6 Conclusion

I had compared these two girls' early adolescence because the comparison illuminates various issues that have to be taken into consideration when assessing the psychological state of an early adolescent: (1) What was the child's psychological state prior to entering puberty? (2) Is the child's emotional environment responsive to the child's expectable internal struggles? (3) Does the child have an opportunity to become part of an idealized other, or a group that could potentially compensate for structural defects related to earlier developmental difficulties?

The comparison between the two young teenagers is instructive in other ways as well. It illustrates that external, potentially traumatic events such as war and social upheavals do not have a direct psychological impact on the child's development.

Both girls lived under difficult circumstances. Anne Frank was exposed to a particularly harsh reality. She lived for 2 years in a secret annex in occupied Holland during WW II. Anne was fully aware of the possible consequences should they be discovered. Still, her diary is mainly filled with the expectable "turmoils" of early adolescence and she had retained the capacity to be joyously responsive to what was happening in her body and in her mind. She remained focused on her studies; studying Greek myth or Algebra did not appear to be irrelevant to her under the circumstances.

Vivienne was not exposed to similar extreme conditions but the social upheavals of the sixties did have an impact on her family's attitudes that could have been significant. One example of this was the parent's attitude regarding sex. While they walked around in the nude, in keeping with the "liberated" views of those times, they also retained a rather puritanical attitude in that sexual matters were not discussed and their presence in their children's lives were not explicitly recognized.

If one can draw some conclusion about the impact of social events on a child's inner life, it is that it is under these circumstances that it becomes obvious how well a child may be "prepared" to meet the challenges of extreme conditions, and how well a family may function as a bulwark that protects the child from the direct impact of external events.

We owe an extraordinary gratitude to young people, who, because of their special gift with words, can tell us about their subjective experiences in a way that many of their peers cannot. Anne and Vivienne, in their young lives and untimely deaths, are benefitting scores of psychotherapists who are eager, but find it difficult to make meaningful emotional contact with their frequently sullen and nonverbal adolescent patients.

Note

1 Dalsimer K: Female adolescent development: A study of The Diary of Anne Frank. Psychoanal. Study Child 37:487–522, 1982.

7 Little Hans

His phobia and his Oedipus complex ("The Analysis of a Phobia in a Five-Year-Old Boy," 1909)

Anna Ornstein

7.1 A historical perspective

The historical significance of the case of Little Hans can best be appreciated when the time of its publication is placed into the context of the evolution of Freud's theory of the neurosis. "The Analysis of a Phobia in a Five-Year-Old Boy" was published in 1909, before Freud postulated an aggressive drive, before the second theory of anxiety and the formulation of the structural theory. In 1905, Freud had finished "The Three Essays on the Theory of Sexuality," in which he suggested that "the motive force" of all neurotic symptoms of later life could be found in the vicissitudes of the sexual instinct and where he postulated that anxiety arose in relation to inadequately discharged libido.

As a researcher, Freud (1909) was eager to find proof for his theory and suggested that "surely there must be a possibility of observing in children at first hand and all the freshness of life the sexual impulses and wishes which we dig out so laboriously in adults from among their own debris ..." (p. 6). It was important for Freud to find evidence of the existence of infantile sexuality and the affects associated with the Oedipus complex because, for him, solving the riddle of the psychoneuroses meant solving the riddle of the workings of the mind.

Placing the Oedipus complex into the center of the psychoneuroses had far-reaching consequences for the evolution of psychoanalytic theory, specifically, in relation to repression as a mental mechanism. Because the development of this crucial psychological mechanism, more than any other, is related to the resolution of the Oedipus complex, once the mechanism of repression was understood, other basic psychoanalytic concepts could be elaborated: infantile amnesia; the theory of psychic trauma and symptom formation; the evolution of primary process thinking into secondary process; and the transition from the pleasure principle to the reality principle.

In view of the centrality of the Oedipus complex to the neuroses, it is of particular importance that it was in relation to Little Hans, whose observation occurred directly, within the child's emotional milieu – a setting that Freud trusted not to interfere with the child's naturally emerging curiosity regarding sexual matters – that Freud asked the direction whence repression sets in: is it from the side of the libido or is it from the side of the environment? This question was the precursor to the one Freud raised later in relation to the superego; how are we to understand the harshness and punitiveness of the superego in cases where the parents are mild mannered and kind? In 1909, Freud answered these questions in terms of the vicissitudes of the sexual libido. Repression set in, he said "because of a somatic … constitutional incapacity of the masturbatory gratification …". Since masturbation provided an unsatisfactory discharge of libido, the very persistence of sexual excitement "at a high intensity" made the establishment of a repression barrier, a psychological necessity. Characteristically for Freud, however, he added that "this question must be left open until fresh experience can come to our assistance" (p. 136).

Indeed, 17 years later, in "Inhibitions, Symptoms, and Anxiety" (Freud, 1926), after the ego has been delineated from the id and the superego recognized as a "gradient within the ego," Freud said that "an instinctual demand after all is not dangerous in itself; it only becomes so inasmuch as it entails a real external danger, the danger of castration" (p. 126).

7.2 Self psychology and the Oedipus complex

A reexamination of Little Hans's phobia cannot be undertaken without exploring the significance of the oedipal phase of development from a self-psychological perspective. The reexamination of the Oedipus complex represented a crucial turning point in the evolution of psychoanalytic self psychology. By including the psychoneuroses in the self-disorders in the broader sense, Kohut (1977) formulated the bipolar self as a supraordinate structure within the psyche.

In order to contrast the traditional view of the Oedipus complex with that in self psychology, it is helpful to consider these differences from the perspective of the three subphases of the oedipal period: (a) the child's readiness to enter the oedipal phase, (b) the actual experiencing of the oedipal passions, and (c) the resolution of the conflict.

7.2.1 The child's readiness to enter the Oedipal phase

We have to remember that Freud's intent with the case report of Little Hans was to trace the neuroses of adults to their genetic roots in childhood rather than to place the vicissitudes of the Oedipus complex into a developmental context. Freud was not at that time concerned with developmental experiences that preceded the oedipal period. Present-day analysts, regardless of their theoretical orientation, would have to take the developmental achievements prior to the oedipal experiences into consideration in order to assess the child's capacity to deal with the affects that are associated with this developmental event. For example, Silverman (1980), recognizing that Freud did not have available at that time the necessary theoretical tools, "completed" the case report by adding to it the "pregenital factors:" Silverman pointed to Hans's "anal-sadistic resentment and jealousy of his mother's babies and baby-making capacity and his phallic wish to urinate into his mother to impregnate her"; and how the child's "submission over the years to frequent enemas contributed to a passive-feminine identification with his mother, and the wish to be impregnated and delivered of babies" (p. 109). And Kohut (1977), from a self-psychological perspective, stated that: "the presence of a firm self is a precondition for the experience of the Oedipus complex" (p. 227).

7.2.2 *The actual experiencing of the Oedipal passions*

The affects associated with the oedipal phase-sexual stirrings and the desire to possess the parent of the opposite sex sexually, competition, jealousy and murderous wishes toward the parent of the same sex, and, most important, castration anxiety – are viewed very differently by traditionalists and self psychologists. In traditional theory, the inherently conflictual nature of the experience and the inevitability of castration anxiety makes repression mandatory, walling off the conflict and enabling the ego to turn to the next developmental phase, latency. Because of its incestuous and murderous content, the walled-off conflict remains burdened by guilt and therefore becomes forever the potential source of a neurosis. This essentially pathological view of a normal developmental phase can best be explained by the fact that Freud had conceptualized the Oedipus complex as this may occur developmentally on the basis of reconstructions from the analyses of adults; the case of Little Hans was to confirm what he already "knew".

Obviously, psychoanalysts have only reconstructed data available for postulating developmental experiences. Kohut too depended on such data for his constructions. His observations, however, led him to a conclusion very different from Freud's. He found that at the end of their analyses, some patients with primary self-disorders developed an oedipal constellation. This he considered to be the positive result of the consolidation of the self the patient had never achieved before. He observed that this "brief oedipal phase is accompanied by a warm glow of joy, a joy that has all the earmarks of an emotionality that accompanies a maturational or developmental achievement" (Kohut, 1977, p. 228). From such clinical observations, Kohut concluded that in normal development, where parents experience joy and pride in the child's developmental achievements, the oedipal phase, rather than being fraught with guilt and anxiety, is experienced joyfully.

In 1977 Kohut still retained the idea that the conflictual aspects of the Oedipus complex are the genetic focus of the development of Guilty Man and of the genesis of the psychoneuroses. His emphasis on parental responsiveness to the child's oedipal experiences, however, indicated a radical shift from the inevitable conflicts created by drive maturation to the potentially pathogenic impact of parental attitudes and responses to this forward move in development. He argued convincingly that the dramatic, conflict-ridden

Oedipus complex of classical analysis, depicting the child's aspirations to be crumbling under the impact of castration fear, is not a primary maturational necessity but rather the result of frequently occurring failures of narcissistically disturbed parents to respond empathically to their oedipal-age children. He called into question the classical conception of the Oedipus complex as a ubiquitous, normal, human experience and posited it as a manifestation of an already pathological phenomenon. He distinguished between a relatively silent and joyful normal developmental phase during which, the child is able to integrate "his libidinal and aggressive strivings" and an Oedipus complex in which normal development becomes derailed, resulting in the formation of an infantile neurosis that may later give rise to a psychoneurosis:

Subsequent to an oedipal phase that is marred by the failure of the parents to respond healthily to their child, a defect in the child's self is set up. Instead of further development of a firmly cohesive self able to feel the glow of healthy pleasure in its affectionate and phase-appropriate sexual functioning and able to employ self-confident assertiveness in the pursuit of goals, we find throughout life a continuing propensity to experience the fragments of love (sexual fantasies) rather than love and the fragments of assertiveness (hostile fantasies) rather than assertiveness and to respond to these experiences –which always include revival of the unhealthy selfobject experiences of childhood – with anxiety [Kohut, 1984 pp. 24–25].

7.2.3 *The resolution of the conflict*

The resolution of the Oedipus complex, which results in the child's identification with the same-sex parent, has particular importance for classical theory. This is the developmental event that finalizes the construction of a repression barrier and the internalization of standards and values; the establishment of the superego as a relatively separate mental agency. Since self psychology views the psyche as an open system, no developmental experience is conceptualized with the same finality as is the resolution of the Oedipus complex in classical theory. The processes of idealization and the need to be mirrored by idealized others continue into adult life; they continue to make a contribution to the development of values and ideals and to the strengthening of the gender-related features of the personality. The ongoing developmental significance of these selfobject experiences can best be appreciated in the need of young adults to be approved and valued by their idealized superiors and in their need to be mirrored in their gender-characteristic attributes in order to feel sexually desirable.

7.3 Comments of the analysis of Little Hans's horse phobia

Only after several readings can one appreciate the value of this detailed case report. The reader can trace the way in which the emergence of new material following interpretations, and the "overcoming of resistances," made the repeated revisions of Freud's understanding of the phobia necessary. We may not agree with his interpretations (and those that were made by the father, independent of Freud's recommendations) and how these may have been responsible for creating the "resistances." But we would still have to admire the consistency with which Freud employed the method of psychoanalysis to arrive at his particular conclusions.

Freud (1909) described Hans as a "cheerful, amiable, active-minded young fellow, whose sexual precocity is correlated to an intellectual precocity" (p. 142). At the time Freud introduced the child to the reader, the boy had already entered the oedipal phase and appeared to be well into the second subphase of his oedipal experiences; he was under the impact of strong affects and expressed a great deal of curiosity. Hans appears to have been a child with a lively intellect who was actively engaged in trying to solve the mysteries of life. He went about this as all children his age do, namely, by first observing his own body and its functions and then trying to make generalizations on the basis of his observations. In keeping with his cognitive development, Hans began to order his experiences and observations about himself and others into categories, such as noting that living things urinate while non-living things do not. A lovely example of this occurred when Hans, at the age of three and three quarters, observed some water being let out of an engine and wanted to know where the engine's "widdler" was. After a while he added thoughtfully, "A dog and a horse have widdlers; a table and a chair haven't" (p. 9)[1]

Hans's father, however – in his eagerness to set Hans "straight" on matters sexual – appears to have interfered with this process of intellectual and emotional mastery. There were a series of instances where the father contradicted Hans regarding the correctness of his observations and instead offered information that the little boy could not fully comprehend and that he experienced as confusing and challenging.

The first and most obvious misinformation related to whether or not women had widdlers. When he observed his mother urinating, Hans asked her if she had a widdler. The mother answered without hesitation that she indeed had a widdler. The father "corrected" the mother and informed Hans that women had no widdlers. Hans first resisted and wondered how little girls (his sister) could urinate; but since his father, in his idealized wisdom, knew "everything," Hans could not simply dismiss such information. This confusing state of affairs appears to have increased his urgency to ask more and more questions.

The father's information to Hans rested on his considering the widdler[2] only as a sexual organ and on his assumption that Hans's curiosity was spurred only by the sexual sensations he experienced in his widdler. Hence, he could not appreciate the child's logic and confirm the validity of his observation, which had established a connection between the act of urination and the need to have an organ to perform such an act. When the father eventually corrected his earlier "explanation" and told Hans that there was a difference between the widdlers of men and women – rather than that one group of people had one and the other did not – Hans's spirits lifted markedly. We have to leave the question open whether this clarification had alleviated the child's castration fears, as Freud assumed, or his spirits had lifted because this clarification coincided with his own observations and his logic was finally validated by his father.

Another remarkable misinformation occurred in relationship to childbirth. After Hans made the correct connection between his mother's moaning in pain, the bloody bath water, and the birth of his sister, he was informed by his father that the baby had been brought by a stork. Because of his very different agenda for the child, this was probably the father's most obvious failure to recognize Hans's extraordinary ability to make meaningful connections between disparate pieces of observations.

In another instance, the father, in his eagerness to "cure" Hans of his castration fear, made an interpretation that must have further thickened the fog in the child's mind. When Hans told his father that he did not want to touch a horse because it might turn around and bite his hand, the father corrected him by saying that he probably meant "widdler" when he said "horse." When the child protested and said that a "widdler doesn't bite," the father could not be convinced and replied: "Perhaps it does though" (p. 30).

Freud knew Hans's parents[3] and considered them to be people who could raise their children without coercion so that the manifestations of infantile sexuality would not suffer undue and premature repression and could therefore be more readily documented. To emphasize the central significance of infantile sexuality and castration anxiety in neurosogenesis and also to undo the influence of his earlier seduction theory, Freud appears not to have taken some obvious parental attitudes into consideration in the genesis of the phobia.[4] The most outstanding example of this omission was the way in which the various castration threats by both parents were not considered to be of pathogenic significance. Freud's argument was that these threats had been going on for about a year before the appearance of the phobia and by the time the child became ill he was "engaged in a struggle to break himself of the habit (of masturbation) that fits in much better with repression and the generation of anxiety" (p. 27). This statement indicates that Freud began to reformulate the theory of anxiety in the course of this analysis. (Indeed, in "Inhibitions, Symptoms and Anxiety," Freud (1926) returned to the discussion of the case for this very reason.) He, however, had not as yet made unconscious guilt responsible for the appearance of the symptom. Rather, at this time it was in relation to masturbation "that the first piece of therapy was interposed" as he eventually concluded that "it was the child's sexual excitement that suddenly changed into anxiety" and agreed with the parents that Hans "was frightened of his own masturbatory indulgences." He advised the parents that in offering Hans this interpretation, they should lay great stress on his affection for his mother, "for that was what he was trying to replace by his fear of horses" (p. 119). One of the most controversial (and contradictory) interpretations relates to the question why horses became the object of Hans's phobia? Answers can only be speculative, for the object of a phobia is over-determined, and each "interpretation" may indeed touch on one or another aspect of this overdetermined choice. This is especially true when a child's shifting, and often contradictory, statements have to be fitted into a particular theoretical orientation. Solomon (1961), for example, was impressed with the pathogenic significance of the tonsillectomy as a confirmation of the child's castration anxiety even though the onset of the phobia predated the tonsillec-tomy by a month. As evidence, Slap cites Hans's frequent references to this event in his fantasies and, most convincingly, for Slap – the fact that after the tonsillectomy, Hans's fear shifted to white horses. After the surgery, Hans feared lying down in the bathtub and became particularly distressed at seeing the black leather straps around the mouth and the eyes of horses.[5] Freud interpreted the child's fear of horses (biting, falling down, "making a row") as a displacement from the hated and therefore feared father – a direct con-sequence of his wish to sexually possess his mother. Many of the child's associations, however, indicated that the horse most likely represented his mother, not his father. Freud briefly considered this possibility but then quickly dismissed it by asking, "What would be the meaning of his being afraid in the evening that a horse would come into his room?" (p. 27). Freud obviously maintained a deep conviction that a horse could only represent a male, and, if the child was afraid, he could only be afraid of his father, not his mother. Nothing could interfere with this conviction even when Hans called the coal-carts and furniture vans the horses were pulling the "stark-box carts," which were obvious references to his pregnant mother (p. 81); or when Hans related his fear of the horse making a row and screaming to his sister's scream-ing "when Mommy whacks her on her bottom and she makes such a row with her screaming" (p. 72).

Along with the oedipal rivalry and hostility, Freud also recognized the child's deep attachment to and love for his father. These, however, had to remain in the background as Freud was pursuing his goal of proving the formulation of infantile neurosis, which he had arrived at from his recon-structions from the analyses of adults. For the same reason, Freud also had to discount the child's repeated assertions of anger at and fear of his mother – most likely responses to the mother's threats of castration[6] and abandonment.[7]

Hans was explicit about his feelings about both his parents. For example, he said to his father: "When you are away, I am afraid you are not coming home." Father: "And have I threatened you I shan't come home?" Hans: "Not you, but Mummy. Mummy told me she won't come back" (pp. 44–45). Or: after Hans came to his father's bed and told him that he was frightened, his father asked: "So you are fond of me and you feel anxious when you're in your bed in the morning? and that's why you come in to me?" Hans: "Yes. Why did you tell me I'm fond of mummy and that's why I am frightened, when I am fond of you?" (pp. 43–44). He also told his father that his fear of watching the men beating the horses with a whip had to do with his wish to beat his mother in retaliation for her threatening to beat him with a carpet beater.

In spite of the child's repeated disagreements with the oedipal interpretations and his continued protestations that he loved his father and feared his mother (which were understood to be resistances), his father continued to make these interpretations since he and Freud "knew better" what the child was supposed to feel. For example, in relation to Hans's reluctance to leave the house, the father said that Hans "sticks to the house from love of his mother, and he is afraid of my going away because of the hostile wishes he nourishes against me" (p. 45).

Hans was brought to Freud only once in the course of the analysis, at which time he told the child that his fear came from being afraid of his father because he was so fond of his mother. Hans disagreed and told Freud that he was not only fond of his mother but of his father as well and that when his father left, he worried that he would not come back.

7.4 A self-psychological interpretation of the phobia

In reexamining the case of Little Hans, we have to raise the following questions: Why did the experience and the resolution of the oedipal phase become problematic for Hans? Why did he develop a phobia in the course of it? From a self-psychological perspective, these questions cannot be answered without considering that the actual threats to the child's physical integrity and the mother's threatening him with abandonment had pathogenic significance.

Anthony (1970) commented on the one-sided view analysts have about the Oedipus complex. Drawing attention to Freud's description of the parents of Little Hans, Anthony wondered why, in spite of observations that child analysts had made on the behavior of parents of oedipal age children, "nevertheless, it is rare in any of these for the analyst's attention to be focused on the parent's reaction" (p. 279). As an example Anthony cites the case of seven-year-old Peter described by Rangell. The mother in this case was described as suffering from anxiety symptoms, "but little more is said about the reactions of the parents – the analysis of the oedipal conflict is confined to the boy" (Anthony, 1970 p. 280).

In his posthumously published book How Does Analysis cure? Kohut (1984) devoted a section to the discussion of castration anxiety, and he returned once more to the developmental significance of the child's oedipal experiences. He did so because of the central role that castration anxiety is supposed to play in both healthy and pathological development. In classical theory, it is castration anxiety that either brings about adequate repression of the infantile conflicts or, when the anxiety is excessive, leaves the repression barrier permeable for the development of a later neurosis.

Kohut distinguished primary and secondary oedipal anxiety. The primary anxiety of the oedipal child, he said, was simply one special instance of the type of anxiety he had described earlier, as "disintegration anxiety" (Kohut, 1977), the experience of which is a profound dread of death and annihilation. This disintegration anxiety occurs when the environment, from an early age on, is fairly consistently unavailable and new challenges repeatedly overtax the child's immature psyche. The second form of anxiety is related specifically to the oedipal phase and "arises in the child when, after the disintegration of the healthy oedipal self, characterized by affectionate and assertive attitudes, the fragmented oedipal self, characterized by sexual and destructive fantasies and impulses, take over (Kohut, 1984, p. 16).

It could be debated, however, whether Hans's phobia was related to castration anxiety or, rather, was the symptomatic manifestation of separation anxiety. I build my case in favor of the latter possibility and suggest that Hans's separation anxiety was an expectable response to his mother's unpredictable attitude as she alternated between overstimulating the child and becoming verbally threatening and punitive with him. These attitudes may well have become accentuated during her pregnancy and after the birth of the new baby. Hans's reaction to his mother's attitude, her overt threats and Hans's murderous wishes toward his little sister, whom he was supposed to love,[8] generated a host of new feelings (anger, fear, and jealousy) in the child, which created conflicts that found a neurotic solution in the phobia.

When Hans first experienced anxiety while out on a walk with the maid, he asked to be taken home because he missed his mother; he did not want to be away from her. This appears to be a straightforward expression of separation anxiety similar to that which emerged when he woke up with anxiety, saying, "When I was asleep I thought you were gone and I bad no Mummy to coax[9] with" (p. 23).

To consider that separation anxiety rather than castration anxiety was responsible for the phobia is not a uniquely self-psychological notion. Bowlby (1973), citing evidence similar to mine, considered the phobia to be related to the child's "anxious attachment" to his mother. More specifically, Bowlby related Hans's fear that a horse would bite him to an incident when Lizzi, a little girl who was staying in a neighboring house, went away and the luggage was taken to the station in a cart pulled by a white horse. Lizzi's father was there and bad warned her not to put her finger to the white horse or it would bite her. "Thus," says Bowlby, "we find that Hans's fear of being bitten by a horse is closely linked in his mind to someone's departure" (p. 286). Fromm (1968) and Garrison (1978) also considered the child's relationship with his mother to be the decisive factor in the development of the phobia. Lindon (1990) is most explicit in this regard. The mother, he says, rather than understanding the child's subjective experiences; was "misattuned, overstimulating, seductive, intrusive, and controlling."

It is interesting that in spite of the many questions raised about Freud's original formulation of the case, it remained the prototypical one for all later psychoanalytic theorizing related to the various forms of phobias. More important, it also remained convincing "evidence" that the oedipal phase of development is fraught with conflicts and inevitably becomes the source of neurosis either in childhood or later in life.

Addressing the question of parental participation in the psychopathology of the oedipal age child, I (Ornstein, 1983) concluded that it may be a historically determined theoretical bias in psychoanalysis that only what is instinctual is considered truly intrapsychic. There is a concern that the recognition of the neurosogenic impact of the environment means the abandonment of an intrapsychic position and a shift to an interpersonal, environmentalist one. The introduction of the concept of the selfobject, however, helped analysts maintain their intrapsychic focus without dismissing the potentially pathogenic impact of the environment not only in the early years of life but in the later phases of development as well.

The many sadistic and sexual features that have been interpreted by classical psychoanalysts as causative of Hans's difficulty in resolving the Oedipus complex would be interpreted in self psychology as secondary phenomena, as breakdown products, related to faulty parental responsiveness to the child's curiosity, his assertiveness, his anger at his mother, and his jealousy of his sister for replacing him in his special position in the family. As Kohut (1984) would say, this was an example where the healthy oedipal self (characterized by affectionate and assertive attitudes) fragmented and sexual and destructive impulses had taken over (p. 16).

Trying to cope with his jealousy and anger toward his mother and his new sibling, Hans looked to his father for closeness and understanding. Although Hans found him very interested in his dreams and fantasies, his father does not seem to have been very empathic to the child's state of mind; he repeatedly negated the child's subjective experiences and his observations of events around him. As a sensitive and bright youngster, Hans correctly perceived his father's interest and continued to "supply" him with information, which he, in turn, with equal eagerness, would take to "the professor." This arrangement appeared to suit both their selfobject needs: Hans needed his father's special investment in him at this time, and his father needed Freud's approval for bringing to him exciting and fresh material about Hans's interest in sexual matters.

What the consequences were for Hans for having to make internal compromises in order to retain a relatively optimal connection with his father and to be able to continue to idealize him is difficult to say. However, observations made on children who grow up with repeated breaches in parental empathy (which are experienced by the children as repeated narcissistic injuries) indicate that such breaches lead to the formation of masochistic and paranoid defenses, which become integrated into the growing psyche as permanent features of the personality (Ornstein, 1981; Ornstein and Ornstein, 1985).

As mentioned earlier in relation to the father's "misinformation," we also have to take into account the state of Hans's cognitive development. Even before the development of language, children begin to be aware of–and be responsive to-the subjectivity of the people around them (Stern, 1985). With the acquisition of language and symbolic play, their need to deal with, and to coordinate, differing views on their observations is greatly expanded. The universe that they are now constructing is subject to the responses they are receiving to their inquiries. "Unlike most actions, the operations always involve a possibility of exchange, of interpersonal and personal coordination, and this cooperative aspect constitute an indispensable condition for the objectivity, internal coherence and universality of these operative structures" (Piaget and Inhelder, 1969, p. 95).

Just as cognitive development, specifically logical thinking, is enhanced by validating children's observations of the world around them, in the same way, recognition and appreciation of their subjective experiences facilitate the thrust toward the development of self-coherence. Children can best achieve these forward moves when their caretakers are able to decenter from their own agendas and when their responses correspond to the child's ability to integrate the information offered. Oedipal-age children need such affirmative responses particularly since this is the age when relatively rapid intellectual, physical, and emotional growth demands an integration of contradictory and divergent affects, needs, and wishes. While being able to retreat safely-and without guilt-into the lap of mother, these children need their parents' delight and validation of their growing ability to perceive the world around them correctly in terms of causal connections between things and events. In this respect, Hans's father failed him repeatedly, but the child's idealization of him never seemed to falter.

7.5 A self-psychological perspective on the resolution of the phobia and further comments on the Oedipal phase of development

In keeping with Freud's preformulated ideas regarding the Oedipus complex, Hans's father wanted to save him from the undue anxiety related to his son's sexual wishes for his mother and help him "face" his true feelings of hate and rivalry toward his father. Being concerned that premature repression of sexual wishes would leave Hans vulnerable to the later development of a neurosis, the father could not be available to the child as a validating and affirming selfobject.

But Hans's disappointment in his father was only temporary. The father's interpretations did not affect the child's idealization of him because the disappointment was related to what the father did rather than who he was (Kohut and Wolf, 1978, p. 417). The father's genuine interest in Hans and his careful attention to the details of his fantasies, in the end, outweighed the impact of the confusion Hans had experienced when his father failed to validate his inner experiences and his observations relative to events swirling inside and around him. His father made him feel that it was desirable to have questions and to ask them, that his son's curiosity pleased and delighted him: his observations may not have been "correct" in his father's opinion, but Hans was valued for making them.

The idealization of the father and the mirroring of the child by the idealized father are selfobject functions that at this phase of development still have important structure-building properties. To be mirrored by the idealized homogenital parent appear to be a special selfobject function that makes crucial contributions to the gender specific features of the child's personality.

This view of the oedipal phase affects our current understanding of the major psychological experiences connected with it. Instead of assuming sexual identification to occur in response to the threat of castration, we have to consider that for a male child to develop a strong "masculine self" he has to be able to idealize his father as a strong and competent male and feel, in turn, affirmed and validated in his own masculine strivings by the idealized father. In other words, we have to distinguish between transmuting internalization of these optimal selfobject functions and identification as it is postulatet by classical analysis. Transmuting internalization occurs when parental selfobject responsiveness is optimal during the oedipal phase of development. This mode of structure building has to be distinguished from identification. Identification, in the context of the Oedipus complex, would have to be considered to be identification with the aggressor, indicating that this is not "the normal" resolution of a normal developmental experience but, rather, that the child's selfassertive competitiveness and need to idealize the homogenital parent had gone awry.

Inasmuch as faulty parental selfobject functions[10] could have pathogenic significance, the Oedipus complex can no longer be considered as inherently neurosogenic because of the strength of the drives or because of the immaturity of the childish ego to deal with the instincts (A. Freud, 1968). Rather, when optimally failing parental selfobject responses are available, the oedipal phase would have to be considered to be that phase in development which makes crucial contributions to the ultimate consolidation of the adult self and provides it with its special features; a self that can "accommodate" needs and wishes that give rise to conflicts, sexual or otherwise and that not only can "tolerate" but welcome strong passions, be these strong sexual feelings or competitive ones. The Oedipus complex, then, instead of being viewed as a childhood illness that has to be "overcome" or "resolved," could be viewed as a period in development that significantly expands the child's growing self.

Just before the phobia disappeared Hans shared two fantasies with his father. Interestingly, both these fantasies were associated with the kind of joyful and triumphant affects that Kohut (1971) described in relation to the oedipal constellations he observed at the end of successfully completed analyses.

The first fantasy was that his father gave him a bigger widdler, one that "was not merely a repetition of the earlier fantasy concerning the plumber and the bath. The new one was a triumphant, wishful fantasy, and with it he overcame his fear of castration." In the second fantasy, he expressed the wish to marry his mother and to have many children by her. The father, instead of being killed, was "promoted" – to a marriage with Hans's grandmother. With this fantasy, both the illness and the analysis came to an appropriate end" (Freud, 1909 pp. 131 and 132).

7.6 The father as the therapist

That the treatment was conducted by the father was considered by Silverman (1980) as having had "inevitable drawbacks." According to Silverman, it must have made it difficult for the father to deal with "Hans's negative oedipal, homosexual longings and … to provide Hans with information about the male's role in copulation and procreation" (pp. 113–114). Silverman also thought that in addition to Freud not having analyzed the preoedipal factors, the father's failure to include the sensation in the testicles as a source of sexual excitement made the analysis incomplete.

Glenn (1980) too considered the treatment by the father to have been unfortunate primarily because "accurate interpretations create the impression that the omniscient parents read the child's mind, thus interfering with his sense of mastery, his sense of reality and eventually, his sense of autonomy" (p. 123).

Freud himself was of a different opinion about the father's role in this treatment process. Freud (1909) felt that

> it was only because the authority of a father and of a physician were united in a single person, and because in him both affectionate care and scientific interest were combined, that it was possible in this one instance to apply the method to a use to which it would not otherwise have lent itself.
>
> [p. 5]

I agree with Freud and would add that in this combination of "affectionate care" and "scientific interest," the affectionate care eventually gained the upper hand. This case history may be an example of treatment in which the content of inappropriate interpretations eventually wore off in the light of a more basic communication in the form of caring and respect for the child's emotional and intellectual growth. For the eventual outcome of "the analysis," it was of special significance that such attitudes were communicated to the son by the father himself.

7.7 Addendum

Kohut (1984) recognized that the pivotal question related to the nature of the Oedipus complex could not be easily settled, and he suggested that "the gap in our knowledge here can only be filled by extensive clinical reports concerning analyses of cases suffering from structural neuroses treated by self psychologically informed analysts" (p. 23). Several analysts have taken up this challenge and reported on their findings (Terman, 1984/85; Ornstein, 1983, 1989). In the two cases that I reported (one male and one female), the male patient's difficulties were related to the area of assertiveness and initiative, while the female patient suffered from an inability to experience her body as "truly feminine." Both patients developed transferences that reactivated the areas of their respective psychopathology. The male patient's yearning for an opportunity for idealization was most poignantly expressed in his regret for having chosen a female analyst – he felt that without experiencing me as a strong and competent male, who, in turn, could appreciate his own newly emerging assertiveness, he could not get well (Ornstein, 1983). The female patient developed an erotized transference and a deep desire to be able to bring a "rapture" on my face that she could experience as the ultimate expression of my pleasure in her beauty and attractiveness (Ornstein, 1989).

In both cases, I postulated that what was revived in these transferences was the "negative Oedipus complex," a constellation that, in classical analysis, has been viewed as a pathological constellation, which, Blos (1979), however, linked, in normal development, to the fate of archaic narcissism. In my view, the transference phenomenon in which idealization and erotization are combined can now be understood as an intense (therefore erotized) need to be merged with the gender attributes of the homogenital parent. These clinical in stances lead me to the conclusion that

> what has traditionally been described as the negative Oedipus complex in the transference, can now be recognized as an effort to resume psychological development at that phase when the child, through phase-appropriate mirroring by the idealized homogenital parent, acquires pride and pleasure in his own "masculinity" or her "femininity".
>
> [Ornstein, 1983, p. 140]

7.8 Summary

This chapter offers a self-psychological perspective on the Oedipus complex and on the origins of Hans's horse phobia. It asserts that the phobia erupted because of the child's separation anxiety, an increasingly insecure attachment to his mother. Although he received confusing and nonvalidating responses from his father, Hans was able to maintain the kind of idealization of his father that is a necessary selfobject experience for the oedipal-age child. From the case history, we know that the phobia disappeared, but we do not know what emotional price the child may have had to pay for remaining in relatively good contact with his father, which helped him become free of the anxiety related to his mother.

Herbert Graf (1972) appears to have retained his idealization of his father. He described him as a man who, in addition to having a doctorate in law, was a formidable scholar of literature and aesthetics … an astute political analyst … and equally at home in philosophy and science and quite capable of talking mathematics with Einstein … He was a universal man but at the same time a true Viennese …

[p. 25]

Though Herbert Graf created the position of a stage director at the Metropolitan Opera House, and he obviously enjoyed the creative aspects of the work, he considered his job to be in the "background" of an opera and himself to be an " invisible man."

Notes

1 A reexamination of Little Hans has to include what we now know about the cognitive development of young children. The sexual curiosity that many parents observe in their children is part of young children's need "to make order" in their now rapidly expanding universe. Singling out sexual curiosity as if sexual matters were the only ones children are curious about may well be related to the fact that adults have more difficulty answering these questions than they do others. Questions related to the genitals and sexual differences appear to have special significance in the minds of adults, and the answers children receive may, at times, be more confusing than illuminating.

The oedipal phase (roughly between three and six or seven years) is the period in cognitive development that falls between the sensorimotor phase and "concrete" operations of thought and interpersonal relations. This is a transition from the sensorimotor phase (when children are dependent on action to orient themselves in their surround) to concrete operations, when they have the ability to build relatively accurate mental images of the world around them. This transition is a lengthy process primarily because to "achieve a systematic mental representation involves constructive processes analogous to those which take place during infancy; namely, the transition from the initial state in which everything is centered on the child's own body and actions to a 'decentered' state in which his body and actions assume their objective relationships with reference to all other objects and events registered in the universe. This decentering, laborious enough on the level of action (where it takes at least eighteen months), is even more difficult on the level of representation, because the preschool child is involved in a much larger and more complex universe than the infant" (Piaget and Inhelder, 1969, p. 94).

2 In the original German, the word used is "wiwi-maker," which is more obviously connected to urination than is widdler, which is an ambiguous term and has more of a sexual connotation. (I am grateful to Dr. Barry Magid for drawing my attention to this distinction.)

3 Hans's father, Max Graf, was an enthusiastic friend of psychoanalysis at that time, and Hans's mother was briefly Freud's patient. The Grafs eventually divorced, and the father became disillusioned with psychoanalysis (Glenn, 1980).

4 In traditional psychoanalytic theory, environmental factors in development and pathogenesis were incorporated into the concept of the complementary series; a term used by Freud to account for the etiology of the neuroses without having to make an either/or choice between endogenous factors (represented by the fixation of libido) and exogenous factors (represented by frustration or overgratification of the instincts). The idea of the complemental series was not clearly

articulated until the *Introductory Lectures* (Freud, 1917), and even afterwards there remained considerable ambiguity as to the role of the environment in relationship to development and pathogenesis. External factors have been recognized as pathogenic mainly in the form of relatively gross physical and mental or emotional deprivation and abuse. Such traumatic childhood experiences have been etiologically linked to severe borderline conditions and to the psychoses, that is, to the nonanalyzable psychological conditions. For these reasons, they have been conceptually carefully delineated from the psychoneuroses (A. Freud, 1968).

5 Black surgical masks were apparently in vogue in Vienna at that time. Freud himself interpreted the black straps as representing the father's mustache – an additional support for the notion that the horse was a displacement from the father.

6 When Hans was three and a half his mother found him with his hands on his penis and told him, "If you do that, I shall send for Dr. A. to cut off your widdler" (p. 8).

7 One evening as he was being put to bed, Hans expressed a wish to sleep with his little friend Mariedl. When his mother told him the little girl would have to stay· with her parents, Hans said that then he would go downstairs to sleep with her. Mother: "You really want to go away from Mummy and sleep downstairs?" Hans: "Oh, I'll come up again in the morning to have breakfast and do number one." Mother: "If you really want to go away from Daddy and Mummy, then take your coat and knickers and – good-bye!" (p. 7).

8 At one point, Hans admitted to his father that he would prefer if Hanna weren't alive. Father: "If you'd rather she weren't alive, you can't be fond of her at all." Hans (assenting): "Hm, well." Father: "That's why you thought when Mummy was giving Hanna her bath, if only she'd let go, Hanna would fall into the water." Hans (taking the father up): "… and die." Father: "And then you would be alone with Mummy. A good boy doesn't wish that sort of thing, though." Hans: "But he may think it."

9 Coax was Hans's expression for cuddle.

10 Kohut (1977) spelled out the various possible responses parents can give to the child's sexuality and competitive, self-assertive behavior. He referred to "optimally failing" rather than "optimally responsive" parents in order to give recognition to the "average, expectable, failures" of parents when confronted with these particular developmental issues in their children (p. 237).

References

Anthony, E. J. (1970), The reaction of parents to the oedipal child. *Parenthood*, ed. E. J. Anthony & T. Benedek. Boston: Little, Brown, pp. 275–288.

Blos, P. (1979), Modifications in the classical psychoanalytic model of adolescence. *Adolescent Psychiatry*, ed. S. Sherman & P. Giovacchini. Chicago: University of Chicago Press, pp. 6–25.

Bowlby, J. (1973), *Attachment and Loss*, Vol. 11. New York: Basic Books.

Freud, A. (1968), Indications and contraindications for child analysis. *The Psychoanalytic Study of the Child*, 23:37–46. New York: International Universities Press.

Freud, S. (1905), *Three Essays on the Theory of Sexuality*. Standard Edition, 7:135–243. London: Hogarth Press, 1953.

Freud, S. (1909), *Analysis of a Phobia in a Five-Year-Old Boy*. Standard Edition, 10:5:5–149. London: Hogarth Press, 1955.

Freud, S. (1917), *Introductory Lectures in Psycho-Analysis*. Standard Edition, 16. London: Hogarth Press, 1963.

Freud, S. (1926) *Inhibitions, symptoms and anxiety*. Standard Edition, 20:87–172. London: Hogarth Press, 1959.

Fromm, E. (1968): The Oedipus complex: Comments on the case of Little Hans. *Contemp. Psychoanal.*, 4:178–188.

Graf, H. (1972), Memoirs of an invisible man. *Opera News*, 36 (1, 2, 3, 4).

Garrison, M. (1978), A new look at Little Hans. *Psychoanal. Rev.*, 65:523–532.

Glenn, J. (1980), Freud's advice to Hans' father: The first supervisory sessions. *Freud And His Patients*. New York: Aronson, pp. 121–143.

Kohut, H. (1971), *The Analysis of the Self*. New York: International Universities Press.

Kohut, H. (1977), *The Restoration of the Self*. New York: International Universities Press.

Kohut, H. (1984), *How Does Analysis Cure?* ed. A. Goldberg & P. Stepansky. Chicago: University of Chicago Press.

Kohut, H. & Wolf, E. (1978), The disorders of the self and their treatment, *The Search for the Self*, Vol. 3, ed. P. Ornstein. 3:359–385 Madison, CT: International Universities Press.

Lindon, J. (1990), Little Hans, his parents and his castration complex: A reassessment. Un-published manuscript.

Ornstein, A. (1981), Self-pathology in childhood. Clinical and developmental consideration. *Psychiatr. Clin. N. Amer.*, 4:435–453.

Ornstein, A. (1983), An idealizing transference of the oedipal phase. *Reflections in Self Psychology*, ed. J. Lichtenberg & S. Kaplan. Hillsdale, NJ: The Analytic Press, pp. 135–161.

Ornstein, A. (1989), Klinische Darstellung. *Selbstpsychologie*. München: Verlag Internationale Psychoanalyse, pp. 43–72.

Ornstein, A. & Ornstein, P. (1985), Parenting as a function of the adult self: A psychoanalytic developmental perspective. *Parental Influences*, ed. E. J. Anthony & G. Pollock. Boston: Little, Brown.

Piaget, J. & Inhelder, B. (1969), *The Psychology of the Child*. New York: Basic Books.

Silverman, M. (1980), A fresh look at Little Hans. *Freud and His Patients*. New York: Aronson, pp. 95–120.

Slap, J. (1961), Little Hans's tonsillectomy. *Psychoanal. Quart.*, 30:259–261.

Stern, D. (1985), *The Interpersonal World of the Infant*. New York: Basic Books.

Terman, D. (1984/85), The self and the Oedipus complex. *The Annual of Psychoanalysis*, 12/13:87–103. New York: International Universities Press.

8 Changing patterns in parenting

Comments on the origin and consequences of unmodified grandiosity

Anna Ornstein

Patterns in childrearing are intimately related to the social-cultural milieu in which family life is embedded. As the smallest social unit, it is the family that transmits the standards and values of society from one generation to the other. No wonder then that the alarming increase in violence among young children in the United States had sparked intense debates in this country regarding "family values." In these debates, many consider the demise of the nuclear family to be at the root of some of the worst mental health problems of our children.

Since it is the family that is responsible for the maintenance of the fabric of civilized society, we ought to be able to define what constitutes a family. *Webster's Dictionary* offers 22 definitions, which indicates that this simple question does not have a simple answer. Even if we had a useful definition for practical and legal purposes, from an emotional perspective, the question of what constitutes a family would be difficult to answer. This is so because in the last 40 years, drastic changes have taken place in the manner in which people congregate, live under the same roof, and share their lives. In spite of these changes, an intact nuclear family is still considered to be the ideal setting in which to raise a child. In reality, because the nuclear family (a breadwinner father, homemaker mother, and two to three children) has been relatively isolated and had little emotional support, it did not provide an ideal setting for childrearing.

From the child's perspective, a more ideal situation existed in the traditional family that best survived in the agricultural society. Children, in this preindustrial family, had a very different position from the one they occupy today. In the agricultural society where every member had to make a contribution to the family's survival and welfare, children were provided with a natural opportunity to develop a sense of their own value. The development of the children's self-esteem was assured because they were expected to perform certain daily chores according to their physical abilities. This may have meant carrying wood for the fire, tending to small animals, or taking grandfather for a walk. In these small but, to the family's welfare, important tasks, children had the opportunity to experience themselves as capable, competent human beings whose existence had value to the social structure in which they lived. Also, importantly, the children were not dependent exclusively on the emotional resources of their mothers and fathers; in these societies, the extended family lived nearby, consisting, at times, of several generations. Obviously, not all was well in this social setting either. In the often small physical quarters and the high level of interdependency between the generations, emotions – envy, jealousy, competition, guilt – could take on murderous proportions and many had wished for the kind of mobility that members of the industrial age families enjoy.

In today's technologically advanced society, many nuclear families are being replaced by single-parent, reconstructed, and foster families. Along with these changes in the structure of the family and at about the same time, we have been witnessing a drastic increase in teen pregnancy, drug and alcohol abuse, and child abuse and abandonment. Most destructive to child development have been situations in which secure attachment is repeatedly interfered with as young children are being moved from one foster home to another. These traumatic experiences affect development in all respects, psychological as well as neurological, creating extreme vulnerabilities in the self. The manifest symptoms related to the vulnerability may take various forms: chronically high levels of anxiety, irritability, delay in speech development, learning disability, depression, and violent temper outbursts. In these cases, the correlation between early childhood experiences and psychopathology, including violent behavior, is not difficult to establish.

However, these are not the only children therapists see because of violent and abusive behavior towards others. Over the last 10 years, I have seen children in psychotherapy with similar complaints, whose parents are anxious about their children's welfare and are heavily invested in them. Rather than suffering the consequences of neglect, abuse, or being emotionally exploited, these children appear to suffer from the consequences of being protected from experiencing frustration of any kind. The parents (frequently high-achieving professionals), in their eagerness not to thwart the development of their children's independence and autonomy, seek their opinion and approval in relation to every detail of the family's life; the children are offered a wide variety of options related to food and bedtime, regardless of their age and ability to make such decisions. As I hope to indicate, this particular parental behavior interferes with the process of idealization, resulting in a clinical picture that is not too different from those created by emotional neglect.

In previous publications, I have described various forms of parental[1] dysfunctions based on failures or partial failures in parental empathy (Ornstein, 1977, 1981; Ornstein and Ornstein, 1985). Among these dysfunctions, I had considered those to be of particular pathognomonic significance in which the child was being "used" as a selfobject for the maintenance of the parents' self-cohesion and/or self-esteem. However, in the cases I am here referring to, the children are not being "used" for the maintenance of the caretakers' self-cohesion and used only to a limited degree for the maintenance of their self-esteem. Rather, these parents' way of relating appears to be linked to their need to secure their children's love and to their anxiety that they will not be regarded by their children as "good parents."

What is the source of the parents' insecurity? What is the reason they fear the loss of their children's love — and how may this pattern in parenting be related to the industrial-technological age in which these families live today? These questions have complex answers; obviously, the various social and personal reasons have to be studied in each case, individually. However, some tentative answers can be articulated in a preliminary manner, even at this time.

The parents of young children today were raised in relatively small nuclear families, and their parents were often emotionally isolated and overwhelmed. The parents of today speak of their desire to be "better parents" than were their own parents, that is, to be more loving and emotionally available than their parents were to them. However, they too are caught in the ambience of their time. The rapid economic upward mobility of the middle class and the access to higher education for women promoted the development of ambitions and ideals that created conflicts with their desire to devote their lives to raising their children. Either for economic reasons or in order to heed the call of their ambitions and ideals, today's parents enter the workforce early in their children's lives; more often than not, the children are cared for by people with whom they are in a monetary, rather than an emotional relationship.

The number of caretakers involved in the children's care creates numerous and hard to resolve conscious and unconscious conflicts for every member in this "parenting unit".[2] Manifestly, it creates a style of parenting that is characterized by material indulgences and frequent and indiscriminate praises for all of their children's activities. Indiscriminate praise is probably the most insidious in its results: the praise and exuberance that the parents exhibit at any manifestation of creativity or accomplishment sets up expectations in the children's minds. Disappointments in these expectations can be profound enough to create self-loathing, depression, and suicidal ideations.

Gifts and praises are "offerings"; they express an unconscious expectation that they will compensate the children for the parents' frequent physical absences and that they will secure the children's affection. The children, perceiving the need for validation and for affection, experience their parents as weak, depriving them of a developmentally crucial experience to be merged with a strong and competent caretaker.

In spite of the obvious differences between the emotional environment of children who grow up with violence and deprivation and children whose parents anxiously anticipate their every wish, the symptoms that these two groups of children develop are remarkably similar: Both groups of children are deficient in their capacity for empathic attunement and they both make use of retaliatory rage to reestablish a disturbed psychological equilibrium — the rage in these cases indicating the vulnerability of the self. Since both groups of children have difficulty adjusting to social situations that require delay and tolerance for the needs of others, they are likely to become symptomatic when they enter group situations, preschool, or kindergarten. Being deficient in their ability to tolerate tension and moderate affect, they are quick to respond aggressively to minimal degrees of frustration. By the time a professional is consulted, the children have acquired the reputation of being "bullies," demanding of attention and readily enraged when frustrated.

8.1 Idealization and the transformation of infantile grandiosity and omnipotence

Kohut, similar to Freud, used concepts (such as idealization and mirroring) to describe analogous experiences that begin early in life and continue in various forms throughout development. An idealized other is an omnipotent other since his/her functions appear to alter the state of the infant's self as if by magic. While during infancy and the toddler years such experiences are primarily related to the physical strength, calmness, and power of the caretaker, later in development, caretakers and others are idealized less for their physical attributes but more because of the values, standards, and ideals that they stand for. Experientially, the two major selfobject experiences (mirroring and idealization) cannot be readily separated; their separation is a matter of emphasis. When we speak of the selfobject experience of being mirrored, the emphasis is on the transformation of the infantile grandiose-exhibitionistic self into a sense of pride and pleasure in who one is. Merger with the idealized caretaker, on the other hand, places the emphasis on the idealized caretaker's selfobject functions and the manner in which these become transmutedly internalized. It is important to emphasize that the "grandiose-exhibitionistic self" and the "idealized parent imago" are hypothetical psychological structures. Infantile grandiosity does not describe the children's manifest behavior. The arrogant and abusive behavior these children exhibit are defensive responses to an enfeebled self —enfeebled because, in the course of development, infantile grandiosity and exhibitionism had not undergone transformation into pride and pleasure in their activities. Underlying the boisterous and abusive behavior is a defective sense of self and low self-esteem.

The inability to feel merged with an idealized caretaker affects various aspects of self-development: (1) It affects the transformation of infantile grandiosity and omnipotence: the child's behavior will not be determined by phase-appropriate self-regard and self-assertion but by infantile grandiosity and exhibitionism. Because the inadequate transformation of archaic grandiosity and omnipotence also impairs the capacity to regulate affects (especially when this is co-determined by biological factors), children respond to any degree of frustration to their sense of entitlement with instantaneous expression of narcissistic rage. (2) The growing child may have to acquire and consolidate values, standards, and ideals more in relation to others than in relation to the primary caretakers. The values thus acquired may be diametrically opposed to the parents' own values and standards. (3) When the process of idealization is interfered with, mirroring experiences also become distorted; missing is the experience of being validated by an idealized other.

Early in life, the acquisition of the capacity to regulate excitation, arousal, stimulation, and tension occurs through idealization of the caretakers' physical strength. There are moments when an adult who picks up an agitated infant and holds his/her tense body firmly while speaking to him in a calm voice, can feel the tension slowly dissipating in the infant's body and can hear the desperate cry becoming a muted whimper. From the infant's perspective, these are merger experiences in which the baby temporarily "borrows" the caretaker's calmness and, with repeated experiences, will make the capacity to regulate tension, his own. Another merger experience is exemplified in situations when a toddler expresses exuberant delight in being picked up and placed on an adult's shoulders. Perched in this position, at this height, the child feels powerful, as if he/she could conquer the world. In this experience, the child is also "using" the adult as an extension of himself, but this time, the merger occurs with the adult's height and physical strength.

In the course of development, caretakers take on a "larger than life" dimension in a child's life in a variety of ways: they are experienced as all-knowing, strong, competent, and dependable; these are the experiences that provide the growing child with a sense of safety even at times when, in reality, the child is in a dangerous situation.[3]

The following clinical vignette represents a case of failed idealization in an intact family.

8.2 Clinical example

The parents of seven-year-old Robert were well intentioned people who were eager not to frustrate their son in any way and provided him with material goods as well as personal attention they themselves may not have received from their own caretakers.

Robert had a four-year-old brother, who at the time of consultation, began to have symptoms very similar to those of Robert. The father had a lucrative wholesale business. The mother had an MBA, but she has not worked since the births of the children; she stayed home to give her children the best possible start in life. Though both parents devoted every free moment of their lives to Robert, the child rarely, if ever, rewarded them with a smile – not that his parents were particularly smiling people; they appeared to endure parenting, rather than to enjoy it.

Robert was a "difficult baby," hard to comfort, easily excited. By the time he was a toddler, his parents became slaves to a strong-willed, angry and "bossy" child; his tyranny over the family had become a great deal worse at the time of his brother's birth. By then, the parents knew that the infant's life might be in danger should Robert ever be left alone with him. Robert and his parents were most distressed by the fact that the children in the neighborhood refused to play with him because he was abusive and controlling of them.

Since it was the mother who called and wanted to see me, I interviewed her first. She told me that she was at her wit's end and was afraid that, in response to the child's provocations, she might seriously hurt him. The incidents she described were truly hair-raising: when Robert did not get his way, he would call her "stupid," "a moron"; he would scream at her, saying that he wished she were dead. He also beat his mother physically; she showed me the black and blue marks on her leg and indentations that the child's teeth had left on her arm. The morning hours were nightmares because Robert refused to get up on time and would throw a temper tantrum when his mother would refuse to dress him and drive him to school. Particularly painful were incidents when he would embarrass his parents in public. In most of these, the sadistic elements of his behavior could hardly be missed. In the initial interviews with the mother, she spent time telling me about her relationship with her own mother. She thought her mother did things for her children for her own aggrandizement; she still experiences her mother as a very insecure woman expecting gratitude and recognition for everything she does for her family. She was determined to be a "better mother" by being unselfish and making herself available to her children at all times.

Lately, she was experiencing her home as if it were her prison. All her friends are out of the home, working at various interesting jobs while she is at home, trying to "prove something." She too had a very fulfilling job before she had children. With considerable shame, she "confessed" that, when things get totally out of hand, she would lock herself into her room and would not care if the children hurt each other. During the last year, she had become depressed, feeling that she was a total failure as a mother. In previous consultations, the parents were advised to lock Robert into his room, but he is now a big boy; she cannot handle him physically. Besides, one time, when she did put him into his room, he pulled down the curtains and destroyed some of the furniture.

The father is a large, somewhat overweight man. He spoke with affection of his boys and was careful not to be critical of his wife, who, he thinks, has been "giving into" the children too much. At this time, he too was bewildered; he tried to "set limits" for the children according to the recommendations of professionals but soon realized that the measures that were recommended did not work. In fact, both parents commented that, after Robert was put into his room or otherwise separated from the family, he tended to become more sullen and more sadistic in his behavior.

The father told me about his own brother, who as a child had the reputation of being "a monster"; Robert's grandmother frequently describes Uncle Harry's behavior of being, in many ways, similar to Robert's. The grandmother herself has a "short fuse"; she too flares up quickly when feeling wronged.

Listening to this family history, I drew the conclusion that Robert's difficulty to regulate his affect, the speed and intensity with which he becomes frustrated when unable to control his environment, may well be related to having been born with a low threshold for stimulation. However, such an inborn, constitutionally determined "handicap" is not written in stone; the pliable nervous system of an infant can be modified by environmental influences. These so-called "difficult children" require caretaking that is mindful of the infant's constitutionally determined temperament and that will compensate for this by providing a low-keyed, calm environment. A child like Robert requires more than ordinary soothing and comforting in order to successfully internalize these particular selfobject functions. Robert's parents, especially the mother, were too anxious to provide such an environment.

My initial meetings with Robert were difficult, as he would frequently refuse to come. However, in the meetings that I did have with him, I could see that this was a very anxious child, vulnerable and shame-prone. At this time in his life, he also carried the heavy burden of considering himself to be "bad," the troublemaker in the family and in his neighborhood. Feeling bad about himself was poorly concealed behind an air of defensive superiority and arrogance. In his play, Robert made great efforts to control my moves and was intolerant of any suggestion I would make. On one occasion, when he ran out of my office and expected me to chase him, it was clear that he was afraid I might not come to fetch him. When I "found" him and said that I was glad I found him and he looked like he was glad also, with a tip of his head, he agreed that he wanted me to come after him. Back in my office, he went directly to the puppets and began to put on a puppet show. I was a willing and eagerly interactive audience. In response to a fight between two puppets, I suggested that the boy who started the fight looked scared and that I could imagine that it scares him too when he cannot control his anger and would hit his mother or teacher. The comment touched off a rage reaction: Robert stopped playing, threw himself into a chair, pulled his legs into his chest, and looked at me with such rage in his eyes, as if he wished to kill me. My first impulse was to move away from him. However, I realized that I was witnessing one of those moments the parents were describing to me and decided to stay close to him and said something comforting to him. At this, Robert suddenly thrust his legs out and, with great force, hit me in the chest with both feet. I took his feet into my hands and holding them so he could not hurt me, I told him he scared me; I could see that what I said made him furious. The wild look in his eyes did not disappear for a while. I also said that I could see that, when he felt reprimanded or corrected, all he could do was to strike out at the person who made him feel bad about himself. I let go of his feet as soon as I sensed his rage subsiding and he could make comfortable eye contact with me. After this episode, I thought Robert would want to leave, but instead, he suggested that we play cards. This was an activity that helped him "restore" himself since he usually won the simple games he would initiate.

This was a fairly classical example of a "play disruption" (Erikson, 1940), a situation that may occur when the therapist fails to respond to the child within the metaphor. Obviously, had I remained within the metaphor, the puppet play could have revealed Robert's anxieties more fully. Instead, by identifying fear as the motive for the puppet's aggressive behavior and then referring to Robert who too may be scared when initiating a fight, I had exposed the very feeling the child was defending against. Though not fully aware of my mistake, I tried to recoup from the disruption by not moving away from him after he hit me in the chest. This helped in repairing the disruption and though the process had lost some ground, Robert indicated his readiness to continue our dialogue when he suggested we play some cards.

In this brief, but emotionally loaded, interaction I witnessed the extent of this child's vulnerability and the rapid ascendency of intense rage once he felt wronged or, as in this case, exposed. I was also concerned with his self-image; thinking of himself as a "bad boy" kept perpetuating the defensively aggressive behavior. In my subsequent conversations with the parents, they told me that Robert frequently said that, because he was bad, everyone would be happier if he were dead.

I met with Robert's parents regularly. As is the case in the treatment of symptomatic children in general, I considered my first therapeutic task to be to assure that the parents do not experience me as critical of them but, rather, someone who understood their plight. Once they felt assured that I understood their disappointment in the child and in themselves, they could make contact with their sadness that they have not been able to enjoy Robert. They could also express their concern that he will grow up to be like Uncle Harry. I told them that I was glad they came for help and that I thought that Robert too could be motivated to change his relationship with them. This was hard for them to believe because Robert never apologized for his behavior.

This took us directly to the discussion of the place that rage and his abusive behavior had in the child's emotional life. Rage made the child feel – as it does everybody-momentarily powerful, but it also scared him and made him feel bad about himself: he was not only an angry, but also an unhappy, child. But, why does Robert feel so easily put down, the parents wondered, why does he not have a better image of himself? After all, they always praised him for everything he did.

I asked them to consider whether he may not have been able to make good use of their praise because his own judgment regarding his various performances may not have corresponded to theirs. Also, by having him decide what he should eat or wear, they may have; inadvertently, denied him the opportunity to look up to them as people who knew best what is good for him. Doing things for him he was able to do for himself deprived the child of developing skills that he could have been proud of; Robert, at age seven, still insisted that his mother dress him and tie his shoes. I also thought that in their eagerness to put their own lives at his service, prevented Robert from feeling respect and consideration for their needs. Obviously, now, in situations when he is expected to consider the needs and wishes of others, he does not understand why the world suddenly stopped revolving around him. It was painful, in particular for the mother, to think that her need to be "an unselfish mother" could have been part of the child's difficulties. In terms of his rage outbursts, I compared the speed and intensity of his rages to a malfunctioning thermostat and said that, very likely, Robert was born with a faulty thermostat.

These conversations with the parents had their expectable ups and downs. On the whole, they helped them consider that the aggressive, bossy behavior was secondary to Robert's feeling emotionally ill-prepared to meet the challenges of the everyday life of a 7-year-old. The father continued to think that the child ought to be made to apologize and that strict punishment eventually will "teach" him what they had failed to teach him earlier in his life. The mother, on the other hand, was better able to appreciate that only by responding to the child's reason for becoming so quickly enraged and not by responding to his manifest behavior alone will Robert be able to think better of himself. The mother became quite skillful in speaking to Robert in a firm voice and not withdrawing from him at times of his temper outbursts. The child's improved behavior encouraged her to continue to monitor her own rages at the child and, in spite of severe testing by Robert, to provide him with firm, but calm, responses that the child so desperately needed.

The family remained in treatment for a little over one year. At the time they terminated, Robert was not completely free of symptoms; he would still easily "lose it," but he stopped abusing his parents and younger brother. Most importantly, there was considerable improvement in his self-image; he was proud of his good grades, and he competed vigorously, but fairly, on the playground.

With progressive development, the clinical picture becomes more complicated. Twinship experiences and the internalization of idealized ideas and values attain developmental significance primarily during the elementary school years and during adolescence. Because these are the times when group affiliations provide opportunities for selfobject experiences outside of the family, children who enter the school years with poorly consolidated selves seek out groups (be these religious, political, or based on shared hostility toward adults in authority) that provide them with an opportunity to "make up" for their developmental needs. Obviously, the most dangerous are group affiliations where group cohesion is attained by shared hostility toward those who are outside of the group. When chronic narcissistic rage provides a group's cohesion, their destructive power does not only affect those outside of the group but also individual members of the group. Since these youngsters, along with poor capacity for affect regulation, also suffer from a sense of worthlessness, the propensity for destructive aggression is increased by the profound disregard for their own safety and survival. When the internalization of values and guiding ideals are also interfered with, the combination of infantile grandiosity, poor affect control, and lack of internalized values becomes a dangerous mixture indeed. Manifestly, the difficulties related to this combination usually peak during adolescence. However, the closer examination of adolescent psychopathology is not included here. In this chapter, I only intended to draw attention to the clinical consequences of childhood experiences in which the process of idealization is interfered with. Such interferences may arise in relation to obvious trauma or in relation to caretakers relating to children in ways that make the child's need to feel merged with a strong, knowledgeable, calm, and confident adult impossible.

8.3 Treatment recommendation

The recommendations for treatment have to be in keeping with our current understanding of the nature of the child's and parents' difficulties. Should the child's indiscriminate aggressive behavior be labeled as "acting out," "limit setting" would be the most likely recommendation to correct the behavior.

Limit setting as a therapeutic measure belongs to a theory in which psychological development was conceptualized in relation to the modification of instinctual drives, and "acting out" behavior was understood as the expression of the unsublimated, unneutralized aggressive drive. Where "id was ego shall be" means that, in ego psychology, limiting the expression of the instinctual drives was considered to be fundamental for progressive development. In this theory, limit setting in the course of development assured the transition from the pleasure to the reality principle with all its implication for change from magical, primary process to logical, secondary process mental functioning. In treating conditions in which "acting out" of aggression would predominate, the recommendation of "limit setting" was in keeping with the theory of the psychopathology.

Once the clinical picture is understood as a problem related to self-development, specifically, to affect regulation, and the acquisition and/ or consolidation of values, standards, and ideals, then the treatment has to be in keeping with this new understanding. However, this would only be a theoretical consideration. More important is the frequently made clinical observation that, rather than improving the behavior, "limit setting" increases the child's aggressive behavior and negative self-perception. This paradoxical response is particularly apparent when limit setting is clone by isolating the child who is in the midst of an aggressive outburst.

There are several reasons why limit setting may contribute to the further deterioration of the child's behavior. Among them is the obvious fact that it does not address the caretakers' own affects. The child's aggressive and provocative behavior creates expectable counteraggression in the caretaker; their need to retaliate can easily be disguised as "limit setting." The need to retaliate may not be manifested by harsh forms of punishment but more subtly, either in applying painful pressure to the child when attempting to hold him/ her or in other, nonverbal ways. The nonverbal aspects of the caretakers' responses are crucial in these situations; much depends on the tone of voice and the firm, but accepting, manner in which a child is being held and spoken to. Stern and his team (1985) had shown convincingly that children pick up parental hesitation, anger, and ambivalence and only respond with changed behavior when the message is completely clear-when the "music" of the communication matches the verbal content. In limit setting, it is not hesitation or ambivalence but veiled hostility and rejection that enter the disciplinary measures. Isolating a child may help cool the caretaker' s own rage reactions and, for this reason, may be helpful; however, as far as the child is concerned, physical isolation reinforces a negative self-image and deepens the child's depression.

Winnicott (1956), who was not a self psychologist but a therapist blessed with extraordinary empathic capacities, did not consider limit setting to be a proper therapeutic response in children with "acting out" and antisocial behavior. He considered "acting out" as a form of communication that had to be understood and responded to accordingly. I recommend that, whenever possible, the caretaker remain in close physical proximity to a child who is overwhelmed with rage and anxiety. A "faulty thermostat" can only be repaired if calming an agitated youngster is provided in the presence of "another" who now, belatedly, provides the needed, calming selfobject responses. For example, my holding Robert's feet firmly in my hands after he had hit me was a form of limit setting. However, by remaining physically close to him and continuing to talk to him in a calm voice, the child did not experience my firmness as punitive and rejecting, but calming.

As in other forms of childhood emotional problems, I recommend child-centered family treatment. In treating a young child, I rely heavily on helping the parents understand the underlying cause of the abusive behavior. The parents have to be helped to appreciate that the child's aggressive behavior in an attempt to regain his sense of power at times when his grandiose and omnipotent attempts to control his environment are destined to fail.

8.4 Discussion and summary

After a cursory review of the changing patterns in parenting in response to changes in the social-cultural milieu in which family life is embedded, I focused on the changes that are currently taking place in the structure of the nuclear family. I argued that violent and abusive behavior in children is not limited to overtly dysfunctional families. The pattern of parenting in these middle-class and intact families is characterized by the parents being indecisive and appearing helpless and weak, rendering them unidealizable by a young child. The case of a young child whose violent and abusive behavior towards members of his family and his peers exemplified the symptoms with which child therapists are confronted with increasing frequency.

I recommended that the treatment of these conditions ought not to be restricted to setting limits to the unacceptable behavior. Rather, the underlying self-disorder has to be addressed, not only by the individual treatment of the child, but by helping the caretakers create an emotional milieu that is therapeutic. By understanding and empathically responding to the parents' confusion, anger and ambivalence when living with a child who abuses them, therapists can help them remain calm in the face of the child's provocations. A calm and firm responsiveness and a genuine appreciation of the child's anxieties, when provided over an extended period, can offer, albeit belatedly, a genuine therapeutic milieu that has to accompany the individual treatment of the child.

Notes

1 I am using *parents* and *caretakers* interchangeably when referring to the emotional milieu created by the significant people in the child's environment. Such an environment may be limited to members of the nuclear family, or it may extend into the school or the community at large.
2 "Parenting unit" refers to a group of people responsible for a child's care. In such a group, even when the mother and father are physically and emotionally available, they are only members of a group of people who are intimately involved in a child's life and are responsible for his/her development.
3 Freud and Burlingham (1943) observed that children who remained in London with their parents and in their familiar surroundings had done better emotionally than children who were separated from their families and lived in the countryside during the war, in spite of the fact that the children in London had to witness the nightly bombings during the blitz.

    Obviously, the decisive factor here was whether or not the children were separated from their parents. However, attachment alone does not explain the almost total absence of anxiety in children who remained with their parents. Rather, I believe that idealized caretakers provide a protective shield against the child experiencing overwhelming anxiety. The shield is created by the child endowing the parents with omnipotent powers to protect them even under circumstances that, in reality, are extremely dangerous.

References

Erikson, E. H. (1940), Studies in the interpretation of play. *Genetic Psychol. Monogr.*, 22:557–671.

Freud, A. & Burlingham, D. (1943), *War and Children*. New York: Medical War Books.

Ornstein, A. (1977), Making contact with the inner world of the child: Towards a theory of psychoanalytic psychotherapy with children. *Comprehens. Psychiat.*, 17:3–26.

Ornstein, A. (1981), Self-pathology in childhood: Clinical and developmental considerations. *Psychiat. Clin. N. Amer.*, 4:435–453.

Ornstein, A. & Ornstein, P. (1985), Parenting as a function of the adult self: A psychoanalytic developmental perspective. In: *Parental Influences: In Health and Disease*, ed. J. Anthony & G. Pollock. Boston: Little Brown and Co.

Stern, D. (1985), *The Interpersonal World of the Infant*. New York: Basic Books, pp. 181–231.

Winnicott, D. (1956), The antisocial tendency. In: *Through Pediatrics to Psychoanalysis*. New York: Basic Books, pp. 306–315.

9 Child-centered family treatment

Conceptual framework and clinical implications

Anna Ornstein

The conceptual framework for the clinical work I shall describe has been derived from Winnicott's *Therapeutic Consultation in Child Psychiatry* (Basic Books, 1971), from the principles underlying the conduct of a *Therapeutic Dialogue* (Ornstein & Ornstein, 1986) and from Heinz Kohut's theory of the *Development of the Self* (1971, 1984).

As you all know, Winnicott's approach to the treatment of children was primarily determined by developmental considerations. As a psychoanalyst, he was mindful of the importance of assessing and thoroughly understanding the inner world of the child (the child's anxieties, mode of defense and adaptation, the child's fantasies and dreams), and – at the same time – he was fully conscious of the impact that the child's environment had on these inner experiences and with that, on the child's progressive development. Combining his developmental considerations with his recognition that children's psyches remained an "open system" (open to pathological as well as therapeutic influences), he had recommended that a therapist ought to aim at "*so that the change he had so achieved can be made use of by the parents and those who are responsible in the immediate social setting*" unblocking the child's progressive maturational processes ... (emphasis mine)

This recommendation meant to me that in order for the individual treatment of children to be effective, the therapist had to do nothing more – but also nothing less – than to remove the obstacles that the child's symptom had set in the way of further growth and development. Symptom removal, however, would constitute only one aspect of the therapist's aims, since "the change that the therapist has so achieved had to be made use of by the parents who are responsible in the immediate social setting." And Winnicott went on to say: "If the child goes away from the therapeutic consultation and *returns to an abnormal family or social situation* then there is no environmental provision of the kind that is needed and that I take for granted. I rely on the 'average expectable emotional environment' to meet and make use of changes that had taken place."

In other words, regardless of how penetrating the therapist's interpretive comments may be, changes in the child can be expected only when the environment is an "average expectable" one: an environment that can be responsive to the child's developmental needs.

But the families that our child patients come from are rarely average and expectable. The changes that had taken place in the manner in which people congregate, live under the same roof and share their lives had changed drastically in the last 60 years. In the midst of these changes, we have been holding on to an image of a "traditional family" which, in reality, now exists only to a rather limited degree.

The traditional family of the agricultural age has not been in existence for quite some time. With the arrival of the Industrial Revolution it has been reduced to the small, relatively isolated "nuclear family." The image of the breadwinner father and homemaker mother and a few children came into being about the middle of the 19th Century and existed for about 100 years, roughly between 1860–1960. In the agricultural era, mothers and fathers worked side by side in the field and there was an extended family that helped in the raising of the children. The children in this agricultural, traditional family had a very different position from the one they have been occupying in the industrial era. In the traditional family, the children acquired their moral and ethical values that would prepare them for a predictable adult existence by the very manner in which the family functioned as a unit. The downing of the Industrial Era changed all these. Young adults left the land and their families of origin; they lost the support of a community and they became dependent on their own resources. Without the support of a community that would nurture their values, goals, and ideals, the nuclear family was doomed to failure. In other words, while the Industrial Revolution created the nuclear family, it also slowly but surely contributed to its demise.

Today, families come in great varieties: single women raising children constitute the largest group. The high number of divorces created a large number of "step-families" with a great number of variation in living arrangements. Lesbian and gay couples raise either adopted children or children conceived by a variety of methods (some lesbians have biological children but that does not mean that they had insemination or else).

In addition, we are no longer satisfied with the overtly "average" appearing environment. We had learned to appreciate the subtle forms of emotional neglect and abuse that children may be exposed to; emotional abuse that the environment itself may be not be aware of.[1] The major and more difficult part of our therapeutic work may not be related to the treatment of the child but to our efforts to create an environment that can not only be "average expectable" but also therapeutic in relation to the symptomatic child.

Many child therapists have become disappointed with the individual treatment of children and turned to "family treatment", that is, they would include whoever constituted the child's emotional environment into the treatment process.

I shall say a few words about why, in my opinion, "family treatment" is not the answer to our therapeutic dilemmas. What I see as a problem in family treatment is that the symptomatic child might not be given an opportunity to be properly assessed diagnostically which may include the need for neurological or psychological examination. Nor is the child given the opportunity to be heard without the presence of others. I believe that the sources of the child's symptomatic behavior can only be ascertained when the therapist and the child-patient are given an opportunity to jointly discover what *this child at this time in his/her life* is experiencing subjectively, that is intrapsychically. In a "family treatment" setting, a child cannot be expected to share his/her feelings freely. Instead, it is a trained child psychotherapist who, in the course of a therapeutic relationship is able to gain insights into the meaning of a young child's symbolic communications (play, drawings). It is the child therapist who ought to be able to identify the child's anxieties, developmental deficits and conflicts underlying the symptomatic behavior.

Another problem related to family treatment is that the time required to effect changes in the dynamics of the family system are much too slow to have a meaningful impact on the progressive development of a symptomatic child. Instead, by identifying the depression and anxiety that underlay and motivate the manifest behavior, the therapist can address those of the child's interactions with the caretakers that most directly affect the child. So, what does such a child-centered family treatment look like?

9.1 The conduct of a diagnostic-therapeutic interview: the therapeutic dialogue

Experienced therapists know that a distinction between a diagnostic and a therapeutic phase exists only in the minds of therapists. As far as the patients are concerned, they want help when they call for help. Winnicott says – and I agree – that this is the time when the child and the caretakers maybe most receptive to our understanding of the nature of their difficulties, even when this understanding has to be, at this early phase, preliminary and tentative. The conflicts in which parents and children have been caught are more likely to become loosened in the early rather than in the later phases of their difficulties with each other. However, such loosening of the pathological interactions depends on the family being able to leave after the first interview, (or certainly after the first few), with the feeling that they have been heard and understood as far as their most urgent current difficulties are concerned.

Here a caveat is necessary: while most of us have little difficulty in being empathic with our child patients and respond to them with acceptance and understanding, this is not an easy task in relationship to the parent(s) and other members of the child's social environment. It is difficult to be accepting and understanding of caretakers who do not exhibit empathy toward the child and whose behavior may continually aggravate the child's already painful inner reality. However, to be judgmental and at times outraged at the parents, will, even in its most disguised form, seriously interfere with our most important therapeutic aim, namely, to help the caretakers recognize the anxiety, depression, or whatever other affects may be responsible for the child's manifest behavior.

Let me re-state: As child therapists listen to the parents' complaints and as they listen and try to comprehend the child's subjective, intrapsychic experiences, they are engaged in an effort to locate that area of the parent-child interactions in which parental attitudes and dysfunctional responses continue to aggravate the child's symptomatic behavior. The etiology, how these problems came about, has to take the back-seat to our concerns regarding the dynamic forces that are currently operative both intrapsychically and interpersonally. We cannot therapize the past – its exploration becomes important insofar as it may illuminate the focal issues that are currently dominating the clinical picture. *What has to become the focus of the therapist's interventions is the area in which the child's psychopathology and dysfunctional parental responses intersect.* As I indicated earlier, the most challenging aspect of this complex, emotionally charged area is the therapist's ability to maintain an empathic listening perspective in relation to the caretakers similar to the one she is maintaining in relation to the child.

Before describing a clinical example in which I hope to demonstrate this rather complex process, I shall make some general comments about the conduct of the diagnostic-therapeutic interview.

In several of our earlier publications (Ornstein & Ornstein 1977, 1984, 1985, 1988) related to the conduct of all forms of psychotherapies – be this focal brief treatment, long term or psychoanalysis – we had described a mode of conversation in which the therapist's responses are tentative and open-ended. We referred to this manner of conversation as a "therapeutic dialogue", or, as you will see in the clinical report, this could also be described as "speaking in the interpretive mode". Speaking in the interpretive mode means to offer explanatory statements that are tentative and open-ended. Such statements can serve as invitations to the patient to correct the therapist's understanding. We found that this mode of conversation is most effective in engaging the patient early and meaningfully in the therapeutic process. A good way to appreciate the influence the therapeutic dialogue has on the process of treatment is to contrast this to the therapist remaining silent for long periods or trying to elicit information by repeated questioning.

A therapeutic dialogue is similar to the manner in which Winnicott engaged a child in a squiggle game. Whether the game was started by the child or by himself, Winnicott would always take the child's lead in guiding him to the area of his conflict. He did not assume to know what it was that the child wanted help with. As he continually, in an on-going way, responded to the child's communications within the metaphor, from time to time he would stop and articulate what he understood the child was trying to tell him. Important in this manner of communication is to make one's comments in such a way that the child can feel free to correct them.

Child-centered family treatment is applicable to the treatment of young children – up to adolescence. Though adolescents require greater degrees of confidentiality and the caretakers cannot be expected to have the same influence as they do in the lives of young children, I find that here too, re-establishing empathic contact between parents and adolescents may be the therapist's most important therapeutic task. Because the importance that groups attain in the lives of adolescents and because of the upheaval that is created by sexual issues, identity formation and issues related to morale and ethical conduct, adolescents are probably the most difficult group of children to treat. I hope we will be able to take up the special issues in the treatment of adolescents in connection with the presentation of a clinical case example tomorrow.

The patient whose treatment I shall here describe was no longer a young child nor quite an adolescent. However, the treatment is a good example of the manner in which the child's difficulties could be integrated into the most central of the family dynamics. As will be seen, it was in the course of my work with the symptomatic child, that my understanding of the child's anxiety helped me understand the most disturbing elements within the family so that these could be therapeutically addressed.

In order to indicate the wide variety of clinical situations, I shall also briefly describe the case of a "parenting child", a boy who took care of his heroine-addicted mother.

Clinical example: Andrea

Andrea was a twelve-year-old girl, the older of two children, her brother nine years old. The father called because the parents became concerned about Andrea's defiant behavior towards both parents but more so towards her mother. The child, he said, refuses any and all requests, regardless of how insignificant. Though I asked that the three of them come in together for the initial interview, father said that the parents preferred to come to the first interview without the child.

The parents were bright and educated people. They spent the first fifteen to twenty minutes giving me various examples of the child's "defiance". The father, in particular, stressed how he tried to reason with the child but nothing he said helped matters. After listening to the manner in which they presented the child's difficulties and the efforts they made to correct her behavior, I said that their emphasis on their efforts made me think that they may be concerned that I might think that they have not been doing their best as parents. The parents responded in very different ways to my comment. Father became incensed that I could even imply that he would, in any way, feel responsible for the child's difficulties. The mother on the other hand, began to cry softly saying that she takes much too much responsibility for Andrea's unhappiness. Holding back tears, she spoke of Andrea having been born after seven years of marriage when the couple no longer expected that they will be able to have any children: "She was the apple of my eye. There was nothing I would not do for her ..." By the time Andrea was school age, mother would do her homework with her regularly, or whatever else the child may have wanted or needed. Mother was now bitter and angry that this is what she is getting for her efforts! Less with a concern as to what this may indicate in terms of the child's level of anxiety and profound sense of insecurity but more as further evidence as to how unreasonable she is, the parents described how Andrea may go up to the teacher's desk as many as fifty times in the course of the day to be told whether the work she was doing was o.k. She does this in spite of the fact that she is an A student. When I commented that they might be concerned that she needs this kind of reassurance, father comparing Andrea to her brother said that Andrea is not very bright and has to work very hard to get good grades but that good grades are very important to her. He thought she becomes "crazy" when she cannot do her work, and angrily demands that her parents help her. We then set up an appointment for me to see Andrea.

Andrea was a pale, soft-spoken youngster, who was not reluctant to share with me the way she had been experiencing her relationship with her parents. She thought that her parents were stricter than the parents of her friends and that she felt that she couldn't do anything right for her mother. No matter what was happening in the home, she was always the one who was blamed. She vividly described her feeling humiliated and very insecure in relationship to her schoolwork as well as socially. She would spend long hours doing her homework but never feeling sure that she got it right. Andrea described incidents of her mother throwing clothes out of the drawer when these are not properly folded. She also described how it used to be in the past between the two of them. Mother used to re-write her papers, at times using words that Andrea did not know the meaning of. She also had to rewrite her homework four or five times because it was not neat enough. She knows that she has provoked her parents lately but she always regrets it afterwards; she loves her parents but is now stuck in a bad situation and doesn't know how to get out of it. I told her that after I spoke to her parents, I began to understand what might have gone wrong and thought I could help her and her parents get "unstuck". One way we could do that would be for the two of us to help her parents understand what it is *she feels* about the situation. It seemed to me that they were upset with her behavior but that they did not know how she felt. She did not like the idea of meeting with her parents; she would have preferred to meet with me alone. I explained to her that indeed, she and I will have some private times together but she (we?) also needed her parents' understanding, without which I alone could not help her enough. We agreed that this one time I shall meet with her parents only but that in the future we will be having some joint meetings.

The follow-up interview is one of the most important aspects of this kind of child centered family treatment. This is the time when the therapist using her insights of the two previous hours has to be able to *translate* the child's subjective experiences to the parents in such a way that it will promote their empathic understanding of the child's emotional life, specifically, the sources of her disturbed and disturbing behavior.

First, I shall tell you how I formulated the focus, where I thought that the child's subjective experiences most directly intersected with the parents' responses to her. For example, when the father described Andrea's "craziness", I could see an acutely panicky child and a father who had no idea what she was experiencing but tried to be helpful the only way he knew, which was to be logical and "reasonable" with her. The mother on the other hand, would become "infected" with the child's anxiety and respond to it by doing the work not only with, but also *for* her, all the while building up not only great resentment but also hatred for the child who so blatantly failed to affirm her. I also thought that the mother's anxiety about the child and her performance in school, could have been responsible for the child's failure to develop a sense of competence causing the anxious, panicky behavior in relation to her schoolwork. Having become intolerant of her anxious and rebellious behavior, the parents were now reprimanding her frequently and kept reminding her what she owed them. In addition, father may well have communicated his conviction to the child that she wasn't bright enough to do the work – attitudes and behavior that continued to undermine the little girl's already very shaky self-esteem.

My job was to find the words that would convey my understanding without being critical of the parents' efforts that would have only increased their guilt and resistance. I had to help them recognize that the child had her *own, internally determined reasons* to behave the way she did. Most importantly, I had to find a way to include into my communication my understanding of *their reasons* for handling the situation the way they did.

When we met, I said to the parents that their description helped me to begin to understand what may be responsible for the child's defiant behavior and that I would like to share with them my thoughts so that they could tell me whether or not I was on the right track. From what they had told me and what I learned from my conversation with Andrea, I said, it seemed that Andrea's defiant behavior might have its roots in a sense of insecurity. I gathered this from their description of her need to check with the teacher as many as fifty times a day whether or not her work was o. k., also how panicky she would become when her parents are not available to help her. Father again said that the problem was that Andrea was not able to think abstractly but the mother picked up on my observation and agreed that Andrea is extremely insecure and wondered where that might come from. I said that at this time it would be difficult for me to say that since the development of self-esteem is a complicated matter. However, on the basis of what they shared with me so far, I thought that her insecurity might well be related to her mother's eagerness in the past to be available to the child in every way she could. This may have made it difficult for her to develop a feeling of competence. I suspected, I said, that her defiance is an expression of her anger for the parents' reluctance to relieve her anxiety related to her work and the way she feels about herself. By refusing to do anything around the house, in a way she is saying that since they are not helping her, she is not going to help them either.

The mother had no difficulty considering the validity of my observation but still fearful that my statement meant that she did something wrong, she said: "Are you saying that I had indulged her, that I should not have done all that I had done for her"? I responded that my comments might have implied that much. However, I had no difficulty understanding why she made herself so available to the child. After all, she had Andrea after seven years of marriage when she gave up hope to have a child; doing things for her was her way of expressing joy of having a child after all. However, we may want to consider that mother's eagerness to do for the child, may have deprived Andrea of opportunities to experience both her successes and her failures as her own. Father, fearful that my comments would upset his wife, entered with the statement that in his opinion the child's behavior had nothing to do with lack of self-confidence. Rather, he felt that Andrea did not have a logical mind and she cannot comprehend abstract ideas. Certainly, I said, I cannot judge Andrea's intelligence and this is something we could assess with the help of testing. However, at this time, I would not exclude the possibility that her level of anxiety may well interfere with her ability to think and to concentrate. My comment did not convince father, who himself has a very logical mind and is obviously placing great stakes into logic and reason.

After a few individual hours with Andrea, we decided that the best would be if she and I could meet with her mother only, without her father. The joint sessions with mother and daughter helped me appreciate the degree of the mother's narcissistic vulnerability. At first, she attacked Andrea for putting the blame on them for her difficulties, saying that was a "cop-out", a way of avoiding responsibility for her actions. Though quietly and a bit hesitantly, Andrea was able to articulate her feelings of anger and her feeling humiliated, anxious and insecure both at home and at school. Hearing this, the mother began to appreciate the emotional pain the child herself was suffering. These meetings turned out to be highly emotional encounters in which mother opened-up more and more and became available to hear the child's genuine desire to be close to her. She could also hear the child's desire to be accepted and valued by her mother and begin to appreciate the fact that the child could hate her with a passion, but also love and admire her.

Mother and daughter grew closer together but father, expectedly, felt left out. Once the four of us could get together, I felt free to share with the father that I could understand that he was protecting mother when he placed all family difficulties on Andrea's shoulder. However, mother and daughter now believe that this made matters between them worse. My explanation was "logical" so it made sense to him. He said that it might be the best way he could help mother and daughter if he did not try to solve their problems; the two of them appeared to be quite able to do so.

Clinical example: Daniel

A young woman, appearing emaciated and haggard brought her 9-year-old son to the clinic. She brought the child to us with a very special request. She asked that we make arrangements for the boy to be taken away from her; she wanted the child to be placed because she loved him and wanted him to have a good life. Living with her, he could only be destroyed, she said. The mother then told us in simple words, that she has been severely addicted to heroine as far as she could remember. She has been through several detoxification programs and she knows that she could never be drug-free. Living as she does could only destroy the most precious thing she has in her life: her son. The mother then described how Daniel has been taking care of her; he would frequently find her in the entrance way to their apartment house where she would lay half comatose. The child would drag the mother's emaciated body up the stairs; make her comfortable until she slept off the booze and whatever else was in her body. With stealing and begging, the boy kept himself and his mother alive.

Daniel was adamant that he did not want to be placed from his mother; he felt responsible for her and knew that she would not live long should he be put into a foster home. This is why he had run back to her when previous attempts were made to place him. Our therapeutic task was to help mother to accept Daniel's need to take care of her; this is what appeared to be his most rewarding source of self-esteem. Daniel knew where to go for help should it become impossible for him to care for his mother. This was not a good solution for the mother but the most realistic arrangements we could suggest for Daniel.

9.2 Concluding remarks

This was a brief summary of a treatment approach in which I made an effort to identify that area of parent-child interactions in which dysfunctional parental responses continued to reinforce – and thereby potentially escalate – the symptomatic child's emotional problems. In such diagnostic-therapeutic interviews, the therapist's task is the early diagnosis, of the child's symptom in depth and the particular vulnerabilities that had interfered with the parents' ability to be in empathic touch with the child's emotional pain. The most challenging aspect of the therapist's task in such a treatment process is to convey her understanding to the parents in such a way that it results in their increasing ability to appreciate the nature of the child's anxieties rather than continue to try to correct the symptomatic behavior directly.

Recognizing the changes that had occurred in the structure of the family, the therapeutic model I described would have to be adapted to those situations in which the biological parents may not constitute the child's emotional environment. In these situations it is a particularly difficult therapeutic task to determine who are currently the most significant people in the child's life. The principle of the treatment approach remains the same: the child's symptomatic behavior is used to recognize those behavior patterns by the environment that are either responsible for, or help maintain the child's symptom. The integration of the child's inner world with the environmental responses still would have to constitute the focus of the therapist's interventions.

Note

1 In contrast to the developmental theory of traditional psychoanalysis where the vicissitudes of the drives (sexual and aggressive) are considered to motivate development, the developmental theory of self psychology holds that infants are born with the need to be mirrored and to have the opportunity to be merged with an idealized other.

10 Early childhood traumata

Adult reorganization

Anna Ornstein

On March 2011 at the Margaret Mahler Symposium "Philadelphia Childhood Losses, Adult Memories" Anna Ornstein gave a presentation about the fate of 6 children who survived as infants without their parents the concentration camp Theresienstadt and who lived as adults an affirmative live without hate.[1]

10.1 Introduction

In collaboration with Sophie Dann, Anna Freud published a remarkable paper in the *Psychoanalytic Study of the Child* in 1951 with the title "An Experiment in Group Upbringing." The paper is a report of the carefully observed behavior of young children who lost both parents and every member of their families before they were one year old. Over the years, this paper went relatively unnoticed by child analysts and developmentalists. When I assigned it to our journal club in the 1970th, questions were raised regarding its relevance to psychoanalytic developmental theory and for the practice of child psychiatry; the objection was that the extreme nature of the traumatic losses the paper described do not have parallels in our civilized world.

In my presentation, I will discuss the findings of this "experiment" because, I believe that today, we can better appreciate the contribution this paper makes to our understanding of the relationship between losses children suffer at an early age and the various forms of attachments they may still be able to make later in life. We may also better recognize the relevance of this "experiment in nature" to the treatment of children whose histories are replete with losses and separations as they are first rejected by their families and then again repeatedly by one foster home after another.

When children who had suffered multiple losses and separations at an early age surprise us with relatively successful adjustment later in life, we explain this unexpected outcome with "resilience." In my view, resilience is a poorly understood concept that had served mainly to safeguard our theories from being questioned when clinical observations contradict our theory- based expectations. Because psychoanalytic theories have been encouraging to follow mainly a pathological trajectory, the theory has not been particularly helpful to understand patients who have been able to withstand extremely traumatic conditions in their childhoods and proceeded to live relatively successful adult lives. I am suggesting that learning about behavior that becomes manifest under extreme conditions reveals properties of the psyche we don't encounter under ordinary, civilized conditions. Learning more about the recovery following the survival of extreme conditions, helps in stepping outside our generally accepted theoretical boxes and recognize alternate ways in which development may be completed.[2]

10.2 The children of Terezin (Theresienstadt)

The word "experiment" in the title of Ms. Freud's paper does not refer to an experiment conducted in a laboratory under artificially controlled conditions. Rather, this experiment consisted of psychoanalytically informed observations that were recorded daily of the behavior of six children under the age of six. As infants, these children were separated from their families and deported to Terezin concentration camp before they were one year old. Here, they were cared for by inmates, exhausted and undernourished women who were periodically transported to Auschwitz. The camp offered little possibility to meet the infants' and toddlers' hygienic and nutritional needs; their physical survival indicates that these infants may have possessed physical and psychological attributes that others who succumbed to these conditions, did not have. There was only meager information available abut them prior to their arrival at Terezin other than that four out of the six were separated from their mothers at birth or soon afterwards.

At the end of the war, the children were 3–4 years old when, as part of a transport of 300 older children, they were airlifted to England. The group of younger children was separated from the older ones and had the extraordinary good fortune of being placed into a nursery cared for by a staff supervised by Miss Freud. In their short lives, the nursery in England was the fifth place where they were cared for by strangers; they were ignorant of the meaning of "family" and had not known anything other than being members of a group.

Reading these carefully prepared reports, one has to admire Ms. Freud's and Dann's restraint of not interfering with the childrens' behavior with a therapeutic intent. No effort was made to "civilize" them in relation to their eating and sleeping behavior which permitted the recording of each child's spontaneous behavior in great detail. This makes the report extremely valuable in tracing the unique and idiosyncratic manner in which each child attempted to resume development within their closely knit group.

The description of the childrens' behavior in the nursery indicates that no one member assumed leadership in this small group; instead, they showed extraordinary sensitivity to each other and were eager to meet each other's needs and wants. Their attachment to each other was such that they could not be separated from each other even for brief periods of time. For example, when on a walk with one member absent because of illness, the children experienced such degrees of separation anxiety that they had to return to the nursery. Most remarkable, and in great contrast to children raised in families, was the absence of envy, jealousy, rivalry and competition among them: "... there was no occasion to urge the children to 'take turns'," reports Ms. Freud, "they did it spontaneously ... they did not compete with each other for favors or recognition" (p. 134). Handing food to others was more important than to feed themselves.

The behavior of these children indicates that in the absence or unreliably available caretaker attachment, the human psyche has the potential to compensate for this by turning for these developmentally needed experiences to available peers. There was only one child, a little girl who became attached to a substitute mother before her arrival in England. She was the only one who experienced jealousy and could be hurtful, at times sadistic, to the other children. This observation alerts us to the close relationship between attachment to a caretaker and what we call "sibling rivalry." Rivalry among siblings is, in reality, rivalry for the caretaker's love and attention: where there is no, or only insecure attachment to an adult, there appears to be no sibling rivalry. Once a child experienced attachment to a caretaker, only then could other children become potential rivals.

In spite of their extreme attachment to each other, individual differences in their personalities and temperaments became manifest and the children were quick to accommodate to each other's peculiarities.[3] In contrast to this deep attachment to their peers, at first, the children were extremely suspicious of adults; they showered them with insults, especially when they failed to meet their demands. Rather than becoming depressed and withdrawn, they remained assertive, insisting on responses that would take their special needs into consideration. Importantly, their insistence that their needs be met was not attributed to unsublimated aggression and untransformed narcissism, rather, it was recognized as self-assertion, a welcome alternative to depressive withdrawal in young children who suffered severe losses and separations at an early age.[4]

At first, these three to four year olds played on an 18 months to 2 year level but made up for this deficit with extreme speed. This was also true for their cognitive development; their language development was delayed that may have been related, to some degree, that they now heard English rather than German or Czech spoken by the adults. Generally, the children were hypersensitive, restless, aggressive toward adults, writes Ms. Freud, but none of them was mentally deficient, delinquent or psychotic.

At the end of the first year when the children began to develop an attachment to a particular adult, their behavior began to change. The change started with the children incorporating the adults into their group: they began to help the adults in their activities like setting and clearing the tables after meals. Now they became possessive and clingy and reacted to the absence of their favorite adult with signs of brief periods of grief. However, this never reached the intensity of the attachment they had to each other and they readily changed the (adult) objects of their affection. Whenever they felt strongly about a particular adult, this would create the expected jealousies and the lessening of the bond between them: they became more competitive with each other and their playful verbal disagreements would become more physical. The children also developed disturbances that Ms. Freud considered essentially neurotic in nature: excessive thumb sucking, and in one case, compulsive masturbation. When in distress, they turned to their own bodies for comfort.

10.3 The Harlow studies

The intensity of the childrens' attachment to each other is reminiscent of the observations made on the relationship between twins but differed from it in its intensity. In the case of the Terezin children, this may be related to the absence or only insecure attachment to parent substitutes, while most twins still enjoy the benefit of some form of attachment to their parents: "Every twin, except those separated at birth, grows up with an object tie with his twin, auxiliary in addition to the primary object tie to his mother and father" (Ablon, S. et al, 1961). I believe Harlow's experiments (1957–1963) on Rhesus monkeys may be closer to the behavior of the Terezin children though here too, we find important differences.

You will remember that when the baby Rhesus monkeys were separated from their mothers at birth and raised on wire mothers or in isolation, they became severely disturbed; they ran around in circle aimlessly, became extremely aggressive and self-mutilating; behavior similar to severely autistic children. When the six month old monkeys that were in isolation, were placed into groups with healthy younger peers, they showed considerable improvements.

Moral considerations could never permit such experiments with human infants.[5] But Rhesus monkeys apart from their primate kinship to man, offer a reasonable experimental substitute because they undergo a relatively long period of development and analogous to the human child, they evidence intimate attachment to their mothers and active social interactions with their age-mates. The most striking piece of observation on the disturbed monkey toddlers was that in socializing with their healthy peers, they developed strong attachments to each other that helped them overcome their aggressive behavior.

The Harlow experiments confirmed the primary significance of the mother-infant attachment but, at the same time, Harlow found compelling evidence that opportunities for *infant-infant interactions under optimal conditions may fully compensate for lack of mothering* at least insofar as peer-peer social interactions are concerned. He went as far as to maintain that it seems possible, even likely, that the infant-mother affectional system is dispensable, whereas the infant-infant affectional system is the sine qua non for later adjustment in all spheres of the monkey's life. The monkey babies who were "treated" by being in a group with their healthy peers did not exhibit any of the maternal deprivation syndromes such as fighting and biting; they appeared to be more mature than the mother-raised babies including their sexual behavior. Harlow placed the critical period in which peer relationships had to be present in order be therapeutically effective between 3–6 months of life. (Harlow & Harlow, 1965). When the 3–4 year old children arrived in England, they were already intensely attached to each other; it is assumed that they were kept together as a group in Terezin.

Could we draw a parallel regarding the observations made on Rhesus monkeys' "cure" by their healthy peers and the Terezin childrens' ability to escape severe emotional disabilities later in life? The parallel, I believe, can go only so far: a fundamental difference between the two situations was that after being separated from their mothers, the monkey infants were either in complete isolation or were placed on wire mothers. In both situations, they were deprived of maternal touch, smell and sound. This was not true for the Terezin babies who remained in a human environment where they were exposed to human sounds and were, at least periodically, cuddled by adults. This difference may be responsible for the difference in the severity of their respective disturbances. However, I maintain that this does not negate the life-saving significance of the infant to infant attachments they had established in the camp and tried to maintain in the nursery in England. While moral prohibition would not permit human infants to be removed from their mothers at birth and be placed into a group situation for experimental purposes, the natural experiment reported by Anna Freud and Sophie Dann met fairly closely these research criteria. This gives the comparison more than passing significance and re-enforces the redeeming potential of peer-to-peer attachment.[6]

10.4 The adult lives of the Terezin children

But the psychological life of a human is far more complicated than that of a Rhesus monkey. While we do not have longitudinal studies on the Terezin children, the book[7] containing the interviews Sarah Moskowitz[8] conducted with them 32–34 years later, offer some insight into their adult lives. The interviews provide only limited insight into the difficulties they encountered during adolescence and the important influence their adoptive parents had on their later development; influences related to the adaptive parents' ability to understand them, their social positions and financial resources. In studying the patterns of their recovery, it is important not to focus exclusively on their infancy *during* the Holocaust but to recognize the *developmental significance* of what their emotional environment offered them *after* their ordeal was over. While their adult lives differed greatly (some were adopted in England, some in the USA, many of the older children went to Palestine), there were a few common features of their personalities that could be related to their shared pasts. They all emphasized the importance of compassion, tolerance, the need to recognize individual differences but not to stand out and to draw attention to oneself. They appeared to struggle with their sense of identity and probably for this reason, many of them (this included the older children as well) desperately wanted to establish some connection to their biological pasts. In most instances this was discouraged by their adaptive parents. Not having any family connections, any relatives who would be looking for them, nobody to confirm their origins, the children were left with an unanswerable question: "If no one really belongs to me, then, to whom do I belong?" They mourned the loss of a more ideal, accomplished self and blamed themselves for not having studied harder and achieved more. In spite of their obvious difficulties, the most striking quality in this diverse group was their affirmation of life; a quality of stubborn durability; they kept hoping, trying to make the best of their lives. There have been no suicides, only one from the older group who came of age in the 60th, became involved with drugs, and another with the law. Moskowitz made the observation that while we all want to live meaningful lives, child-survivors appear to feel still a deeper call not to live life trivially; they created meaning in their lives by finding ways to be helpful to others.

One of the groups more fundamental motivation was to have a family of their own. We have to wonder: what kind of parents have they become? Seemingly, all who have become parents cared for their children with a great sense of responsibility. But can people with this history become emotionally available, empathic parents? Research has been indicating that babies of depressed and emotionally disengaged mothers (as we assume the caretakers of these infants to have been in Terezin), also become depressed and disengaged with their own children. And there are other more subtle but important developmental factors to consider: Infant research helped us appreciate the developmental significance of mutual regulation, failure of which results in the infant becoming too dependent on self-regulation and burdened by the management of negative affects which then gets carried into interaction with the next generation (Beebe, B. & Lachmann, F., 2003). We also learned a great deal from the study of insecure and disorganized attachment patterns and their maladaptive consequences for further development (Main and Solomon, 1990); Lyons-Ruth, K., 1991).

Trying to understand the exceptions to these generally accepted expectations, I find Fonagy's observation of interest. Fonagy (1993) draws attention to the importance of the caretaker's self-reflective capacity: mothers who had experienced deprivation, neglect or abuse in their childhoods are less likely to transmit these to their children through insecure attachment if these mothers developed a high self-reflective capacity. In other words, this observation would indicate that a caretaker's traumatic experiences are less significant than how well these experiences have been processed.[9]

10.5 Attachment, mourning and "going on living"

One way to asses these childrens' emotional maturity is to consider whether or not as adults they were able to engage the arduous emotional task of mourning? Bowlby (1963) whose work has been groundbreaking regarding loss, attachment and mourning, spelled out the behavioral consequences of loss in early childhood. "The thesis I am advancing" he wrote, "is twofold: first, that once a child has formed a tie to a mother figure, which ordinarily occurs by the middle of the first year, its rapture leads to separation anxiety and grief and sets in train processes of mourning; secondly, that in the early years of life these mourning processes not infrequently take a course unfavorable to future personality development and thereby predispose to psychiatric illness." (p. 500). In other words, *the ability to mourn presupposes the presence of some form of attachment*, be it secure, insecure, avoidant or disorganized. And since the ability to mourn (acceptance of the loss and the gradual internalization of the lost object) is not restricted to the loss of significant others but it is also essential in overcoming everyday separations and disappointments, this mental function plays a central role in the mature human psyche.

We get only a limited view of their ability to mourn from the interviews with Moskowitz. We can see it in Jack who returned to Vienna looking for his parents' original home, and who insisted in naming his daughter after his biological mother; Jack cried openly and with relief as he spoke about the losses in his life. There is a hint of this in Berli whose mourning may have been facilitated by living with his survivor parents who were also his relatives. Judit expressed her mourning by caring for the widows who lost their husbands in the various wars in Israel. In general, their pattern of mourning does not appear to be different from other survivors who had lost their whole families and communities later in their lives (Ornstein, A. 2010).

The challenge for us today is to understand and to explain these childrens' *ability* to make use of their post-war emotional environments and to be able to place such high value on compassionate and caring behavior. In trying to answer these questions, I will use the explanatory power of psychoanalytic self psychology.

As you know, Kohut formulated the theory of self by using his observations regarding his patients' narcissistic (later to be called selfobject) transferences. He used the same method as did Freud who built the edifice of his theory on the basis of transferences he had observed. The fundamental difference between the two theories is that while Freud's observation of unresolved, drive-related conflicts led him to the recognition of the *repetition of these conflicts* in the transference, Kohut (1971) on the other hand, drew attention to the *reactivation of developmental needs* in the transference that were unmet by his patients' childhood environment. In my view, the traditional psychoanalytic emphasis on transference as *repetition* obscured the patient's expectations and hopes to get what they needed for the completion of their development in the analytic-therapeutic situation. In an analysis guided by self psychology on the other hand, the focus is on the reactivated developmental needs for recognition, validation and the need to be merged with the idealized analyst. Clearly, the reactivation of these needs in the transference has to be "untangled" from the layers of defenses that have become established in response to their repeated frustration over a life time (A. Ornstein, 1991). Important in our consideration in relation to the fate of the Terezin children is the observation that selfobject transferences do not become activated only in a therapeutic–analytic relationship. Throughout life, children as well as adults attempt to extract the developmentally needed responses from their environment. Once the Terezin children were in an emotionally reliable environment, they were able to utilize the accepting and empathic responses of the adults around them indicating that the psyche remains an open system and that it continues to be able to utilize such responses for belated structure building.

Related to the possibility of belated structure building is Emde's (1991) work in which he presented evidence that "positive emotions activate and guide behavior and are separately organized from negative emotions and *are often associated with incentive emotion, i.e. expectations about sought-after environmental stimuli* (pp. 29–30). Similarly, Folkman and Moskowitz (2000) found that positive affect can concur with distress during a given period and that this can affect and increase cognitive and emotional flexibility. These findings give support to Kohut's observation that neurotic difficulties do not necessarily interfere with living a productive and creative life.

10.6 Memory and psychic continuity

In the development of the core self, says Daniel Stern (1985), it is memory that integrates the diverse features of lived experience. In psychoanalysis we think of memory either as consciously remembered experiences (the narrow way) or as experiences that are "remembered" in the body, in repetitive actions or other symptomatic forms of behavior. Fragments of memories that induce emotional trauma are different from ordinary memories, writes Daniel Schachter (1996), they are unusually accurate and appear to depend on special encoding mechanisms in the brain. There are an increasing number of PET (positron emission tomography) studies that highlight those areas of the brain that are involved in the encoding of traces of traumatic memories. This may explain the flashbacks, the nightmares and resistance to treatment in cases of chronic PTSD, especially prevalent among combat veterans.

None of the adult child-survivors had any memory of Terezin. We have to assume that their experiences in the camp had undergone infantile amnesia.[10] We have no knowledge of somatic disturbances that could constitute the legacy of their traumatic pasts, which, naturally, does not mean that such were not present. To learn about the ability to recall the memories of this particular traumatic past, we have to turn to an older group of child survivors of the Holocaust.

I had the opportunity to comment a roundtable discussion of four psycho-analysts who, as children, were hidden during WWII. (A. Ornstein, 2007). All four were less than eight years old; the youngest was four when they experienced dislocations, disruptions and terror. However, in contrast to the Terezin children, these children had their mothers with them through most of their ordeals.

For adults who survived a traumatic past, the recall of memories is a par-ticularly difficult task because vivid as these might be, they tend to return in confusing images. However, for Holocaust survivors, each fragment of memory is precious as they serve as nuclei for the integration of their life's story into a coherent whole. Regardless of how painful these memories may be, they facilitate an ongoing mourning process; grief provides a sense of con-nection to the past; a sense of continuity that reinforces one's sense of iden-tity. For child survivors, the problem arose after the war when the adults, be these their adoptive or their biological parents, or their psychoanalysts, failed to appreciate the help they needed in reconstructing the fragments of their memories. Autobiographical memory, says Leavy (1980) can only be recon-structed by dialogue, never through introspection, everything that is "remem-bered" is the product of integration of the past with the present. Robert Krell (1993), a child psychiatrist and child survivor himself, who was separated from his family and placed with a gentile family when he was two years old, writes that when he was told that he was too young to remember, he would become angry, feeling that such responses robbed him from an important aspect of his core identity. One can well understand the parents' wish to spare their children these painful memories, however, it is more difficult to under-stand the experiences that many child- as well as adult survivors report about their treatment experiences. Among the four psychoanalysts who are child-survivors, only one felt understood by his analyst, the others thought, that their analysts' difficulty was related to their ignorance about the Holocaust. I don't think so. Rather, I believe, it was most likely related to what psychoan-alytic theory prescribed as the proper conduct of an analysis in the 1960th and 70th. Long silences were supposed to promote spontaneously emerging trans-ferences and childhood memories. This strictly "one person psychology" has only been slowly replaced by the dyadic nature of the analytic process. And, still, we find that what may interfere with analysts' efforts to empathically immerse themselves into their patients' experiences is that what they hear is not based on common experiences or anything that could be readily ima-gined. Survivors of trauma have every reason to expect that their story will evoke fear, confusion, horror and disbelief and in an effort to protect them-selves from these potentially disorganizing affects, analysts and therapists may resort to generalizations, quick explanations or praise for the survivor's heroism and special qualities. Such responses however make it impossible for survivors to proceed and the affects associated with the traumatic memories may never, or only peripherally, enter the dialogue. In my view, integration of traumatic memories into the flow of one's life's narrative is best achieved through a therapeutic dialogue in which the articulation of images and the reconstruction of memory fragments are undertaken jointly by patient and analyst. This may require that survivors "educate" their analysts regarding the subject of which they speak and that analysts allow themselves to be educated (Ornstein, A. 1986).

10.7 Summary

Based on observations made on young children who as infants were separated from their mothers at birth and cared for in a concentration camp by inmates who were periodically deported, I suggested that the examination of the emotional survival of these children could open up new questions regarding our psychoanalytic developmental theories. The paper raises questions as to the place that infant to infant attachment has in development when adult-infant attachment is absent or only I unreliably present. Peer to peer attachment may explain the particular importance the Terezin children placed on compassion and caring in their adult lives. I suspect that such alternate avenues for development are not uncommon even under ordinary, civilized conditions and would need to be studied more systematically. In addition, conceptualizing the psyche as an open system so that it is available to accepting, validating selfobject responses later in life, may not only help explain the frequently made observation that children with early losses and separation are still able to live satisfactory adult lives, but also their ability to become competent and responsive parents.

This emphasis on the potential to resume development and to recover sufficiently to be able to mourn their lost childhoods, does not deny the fact that among the ones who had "made it," there are many who remained overwhelmed by grief and rage and live without the capacity to enjoy the blessings of everyday life. The "awesome task faced by child survivors" wrote Moskowitz and Krell (1990) "included the reconstruction of a terrible past into a sensible present. In order to imbue life with meaning, a sense of continuous sense had to be derived from the most fragile and discontinuous beginnings" (1990).

Notes

1 A revised version was published under the title: *Childhood Losses, Adult Memories* in Akhtar, S. (Ed.) (2012): The Mother and Her Child. Plymouth UK (Jason Aronson) pp. 107–120.
2 It is helpful to remember that the study of extreme situations had served psychoanalytic developmental theory well in the past. Modern infant research is deeply indebted to Rene Spitz's studies on hospitalism, a study that provided insight into observations made on hospitalized and institutionalized infants and children. By comparing the development of infants in four different settings, Spitz was able to confirm the frequently made observation that infants who spent their early years in institutions had a much higher rate of morbidity and mortality than infants raised in a family setting. Once these randomly made observations could be

verified by a systematically controlled study, *the maternal deprivation syndrome* became the foundation of modern attachment research.

3 Miriam, a pretty red haired child behaved toward the other children as if she were a superior human being and let herself be spoiled by them. But she did not control or govern the group. Rather, she needed a special kind of attention and the other children sensed this and did their best to fulfill it. For example, Miriam liked to sit in a comfortable chair but she rarely had to fetch the chair for herself, the other children brought it for her to the sandbox, to the garden, wherever she happened to be.

4 A personal note: my mother who, at age 46 survived various concentration camps, was the head of an orphanage near Budapest after the war. She and her devoted staff took care of 40 orphaned Jewish children mostly of latency age and early adolescence. Here, I witnessed not only the childrens' remarkable recovery but my mother's as well. Being called "Ima" and appreciated and loved by the children for creating a relaxed, home-like atmosphere, she began the hard work of mourning the loss of her two sons and her husband.

5 Chances are that today Harlow could not conduct such investigations on monkeys either. It was following the extreme physical and psychological damage he inflicted on these baby monkeys that parameters were set to animal studies.

6 In a previous publication (A. Ornstein, 1985) I reported that after family members were separated from each other, inmates of concentration camps formed small social groups that functioned as a substitute family that facilitated adaptation to the extreme conditions of camp life. There was fierce loyalty and much sacrifice within the groups while people outside of the group were viewed with suspicion.

7 Love Despite of Hate Child, Survivors of the Holocaust and Their Adult Lives Schocken Books, 1983.

8 Child therapist and Professor of Human Development, California State University

9 Gadi was adapted at age of 4½. He described a difficult adjustment; he threw temper tantrums and at one time, tried to walk back to England. His physician father wished he would become a doctor but he preferred teaching. He had a masters degree in education and was teaching world culture and political history. When asked about his values, he enumerated them: privacy, individualism, education, creature comforts, art, human rights, and idealism. He was teaching his students how isolation leads to the lack of understanding and lack of understanding leads to prejudice. When teaching, he tells the students of his own life how he was left on a park bench when he was 3 weeks old, taken to a convent and then put into a concentration camp. Once he found out that his parents lived in Berlin, he wanted to see the place. Gadi did not get married but lived with a woman and was taking care of his dying aunt. He did not like psychoanalysis (his aunt was one), they ask too many questions, he said. His early memory was getting lost in an airport and being found. He was receiving chemotherapy at the time of the interview and died shortly after.

Moskowitz described Bella as radiating vitality. She was adapted at age 5 and did not remember anyone caring for her prior to that time. She was determined to find out about her biological past but was repeatedly discouraged. At the time of the interview, Bella took care of the finances of an Art Gallery. When asked how she regards herself, she said: "Jewish in thought, extremely so.... I have been very interested in the history from biblical times right through. I feel that having Jewish identity *is* learning about the history of Judaism and the Jewish people. That way one had continuity and I suppose in a way that substituted for my lack of family: the whole Jewish history and race was my family." Bella was not happy with her adaptive family and left them during her adolescence, so she made Jewish history and the Jewish people into her family. Referring to her childhood, she remembered having been self-sufficient "even in those days." She remembered that in the nursery she did not wet the bed, "didn't have bottles or nappies or anything like that" ... She had no memory of Terezin. Though she is not close to her adaptive parents, she encourages the relationship between them and her children. She feels that her children can give to her parents what she could not give to them. She didn't tell her children about her past but plans to do so when they are older. She talked about hate being a terrible thing and was of the opinion that while what happened in Germany should never be forgotten, "in the main, there should not be too much bitterness because the new German generation cannot be held responsible for the faults of their parents and grandparents." She was rebellious during adolescence but no longer: "I am just myself and what I made of myself." When Moskowitz praised her, Bella laughed and said: "It's has been a lot of hard work. But I learned a lot from my experiences, and I learn all the time ... Having gone through all this, I can sympathize and understand other people better ... lot of people come to me and I can spend hours listening to them ... if you love people enough, they will love you and that other people matter." When something troubles her, she turns to her husband. Sometimes, she thinks, she should have been a psychoanalyst. When asked to help with adoptions she refused and said that "if children come from good group homes where they have the companionship of other children, I think sometimes they are better off there than being isolated individually into families that don't really know how to cope with them."

Berli had a troubled adolescence and could not join his adoptive parents in the USA until he was 15 years old. He feels regret about his behavior, knowing that the people in England were trying to be helpful. He was married briefly and, at the time of the interview, he lived with his adoptive parents, survivors themselves who were his biological relatives. Berli volunteered for Vietnam in 1968. There he regularly visited orphanages and distributed food and gifts to the children. He says: "I figured I didn't have no mother and father to guide me, so I figure these kids could use some help." He loved the way the children would swarm around him ...

Judit married to a well-to-do dentist who welcomed the idea that people like Judit will be given a chance to tell their stories. Her home was full of people, warmth and sunlight and with the sounds of her children. Judit visits war widows in Israel and helps organize trips for them. She feels she has to give because, she says: "I have so much!"

Jack found out that his family came from Vienna at the time he needed some papers for his marriage. It was also then that he found out that he was in a concentration camp for 2 and 1/2 years. After many years of agony, he felt that he had to go to Vienna and said to Sara Moskowitz: "While I am living I've got a lot of seeing to do, for my parents who died, live through me, and I have got to see for them as well." In spite of his adaptive parents' objections, he was determined to name his daughter after his mother whom he never knew. Looking into his daughter's face, he mused: "This is as close as I will ever come to see a picture of my mother." There is deep sadness in these words, and Jack cries freely while being interviewed. Jack, like all survivors of similar tragedies, lives with a life-long regret of having been deprived of the most essential thing in life, a mother.

Leah was separated from the group because of an infection was in psychological treatment until age 18 and eventually found "salvation" in Christianity. She is still struggling with various phobias but she too is married and is very devoted to her husband and four children.

10 "What determines the unavailability of individual memories before a certain age is not a repression barrier against infantile instinctual impulses but the immaturity of the cognitive-perceptual system which is not sufficiently advanced for individual episodes to be encoded (D. Stern, 1985, p. 98n).

References

Ablon, S., Harrison, A.M., Valenstein, A.F., & Gifford, S. (1986): Special Solution to Phallic-Aggressive Conflicts in Male Twins, *Psa. S. Child* 4:239–257

Beebe, B. & Lachmann, F. (2003): The Relational Turn in Psychoanalysis: A Dyadic Systems's View from Infant Research, Contemporary *Psychoanalysis*, 39:579–409

Emde, R. (1991): Positive Emotions for Psychoanalytic Theory: surprises from infancy research and new directions, *JAPA* 39S:5–44

Folkman, S. & Moskowitz, J. (2000): Positive Affect and the Other Side of Coping, *American Psychologist* 55:647–654

Fonagy, P. (1993): Psychoanalytic and Empirical Approaches to Developmental Psychopathology: an object relational perspective. *JAPA* 41S:245–260

Freud, A. & Dann, S. (1951): An Experiment in Group Upbringing, *Psa. S. Child* 6:127–168

Harlow, H. F. & Harlow, M.K. (1965): The Affectional Systems in: *Behavior in Non-Human Primates* (eds.) Schrier, A.M. Harlow, H. F. and Stollowitz, F. Academic Press, New York

Kohut, H. (1971): *The Analysis of the Self*, Int. U. Press, New York

Krell, R. (1993): Child Survivors of the Holocaust—Strategies of Adaptation, *Can. J. Psychiatry* 38:384–389

Leavy, S. (1980): *The Psychoanalytic Dialogue*, Yale U. Press, New Haven, CT

Lyons-Ruth, K. et al. (1991): Disorganized Attachment Behavior in Infancy; short term stability, maternal and infant correlates and risk-related subtypes *Developmental Psycho-pathology* 3:397–412

Main, M. & Solomon, J. (1990): Procedures for Identifying Infants Disorganized/Disoriented during Ainsworth Strange Situation, In: *Attachment in Pre-school years: Theory, Research and Intervention* (eds.) Greenberg, M.T. and Cichetti, D. Chicago U. Press, Chicago, Ill. Pp. 121–160

Moskowitz, S. (1983): *Love Despite Hate, Child Survivors of the Holocaust and Their Adult Lives*, Schocken Books, New York

Moskowiyz, S. & Krell, R. (1993): Child Survivors of the Holocaust: Psychological Adaptations to Survival, *Isr. J. Psychiatry* 27:81–91

Ornstein, A. (1985): Survival and Recovery *Psa. Inquiry* 5(1):99–130

Ornstein, A. (1991): The Dread to Repeat and the New Beginning: Comments on the Working Through Process in Psychoanalysis, *JAPA* 39:377–398

Ornstein, A. (2007): Roundtable Conversation of Child Survivors of the Holocaust, *Psycho analytic Perspectives* 5:5–12

Ornstein, A. (1986): The Holocaust: Reconstruction and the Establishment of Psychic Continuity, in: *The Reconstruction of Trauma; its significance in clinical work* (ed. A. Rorhstein), Workshop Series of the Am. Psa. Assn. Monograph 2, pp. 171–181

Ornstein, A. (2010): The Missing Tombstone; Reflections on Mourning and Creativity, *JAPA* 58 (4):631–648

Schachter, D. (1996): *Searching for Memory; the brain, the mind, and the past*, Basic Books, New York

Stern, D.N. (1985): *The Interpersonal World of the Infant* Basic Books, New York

Spitz, R.A. (1945): Hospitalism – An inquiry into the Genesis of Psychiatric Conditions in Early Childhood *Psa. S. Child* 1:53–74

11 Closing remarks

Eva Rass

In 1976 Anna Ornstein entered the scientific community with her essay "Making contact with the inner world of the child: Toward a theory of psychoanalytic psychotherapy with children." This first publication can be compared to an overture of an opera as this ground breaking and forward-thinking work contained many important elements which illuminated not only theoretically but also clinically Anna Ornstein's basic lines of thought. While integrating the theoretical concept of Heinz Kohut's analytic self psychology with her personal and professional experience, she developed a new therapeutic conceptualization. This conceptualization that differs from traditional child psychoanalysis has been developed further and expanded.

Already in this early work, Anna Ornstein described theoretically and clinically the different intra-psychological and inter-personal relationship patterns within a family system and her findings and her approach fits seamlessly and without dissonance with the results of modern infant and attachment research, neurobiology, and affect regulation theory. Similarly to Winnicott, Ornstein saw the life span as a course of developmental tasks for which the environment should provide a suitable framework. Within this conceptualization, stagnation, disease, or sickness signalize that the developmental path is interrupted with obstacles and is adversely affected. Again in agreement with Winnicott, Ornstein never defined a child as an isolated human being but as a part of the family dynamic and therefore the treatment process should always have this dynamic in mind working in the triad: parents, child, and therapist.

An intense therapeutic bond between patient and therapist is sometimes necessary for entering developmental realms when dissonances within the family relationship system aggravate or hinder psychic internal processes. But it is vital to encourage the family environment to integrate the newly developed elements into the family dynamic. With this approach Anna Ornstein developed a new perspective for psychoanalytic child treatment which differs clearly from frequently practiced psychoanalytic treatment with children and adolescents with its emphasis on transference and countertransference processes. Based on analytic self psychology that considers child development and parenting as a self-selfobject relationship, she used the ideas of modern attachment and affect regulation theory within her psychodynamic and treatment concepts very early. Ornstein realized the chances and failures within the family field, the activated selfobject and attachment needs with the privation and arousal which requires consistent regulation, soothing, and satisfaction.

In case of a family emotional failure, the therapeutic relationship can be used to recognize psychic disturbances that can facilitate supporting interventions, however, the therapist will never take the place of a primary attachment caregiver. If the therapist did become an attachment figure, this could end in a severe frustration as an attachment relationship is based on continuity and in case of termination of therapy this would result in a relationship break up. These findings and professional experiences therefore led to Anna Ornstein's conceptualization of a psychodynamic child centered treatment where the child is seen as a member of the family group and therefore the treatment approaches the group and the embedded relationship pattern from the perspective of the growing and burdened child.

The shown writings differentiate this approach theoretically and clinically, and show and the given opportunities to get the parents in the "therapeutic boat". Their cooperation and possible enhancement of the environment can build a therapeutic milieu around the burdened child in order to facilitate a reorganization of the child's inner world. This therapeutic milieu which is also described as "secure basis" within attachment theory forms a basis for a more sensitive and appropriately responsive caregiving structural growth and expansion.

Through working out the importance of the selfobject function of the adults it becomes clear that the growth process through treatment is not only significant for the child but also for the parents. This can only be achieved if the parents are supported to put all the growth prohibiting obstacles aside that are deeply embedded into their own development as these obstacles are otherwise transferred trans-generationally into the development process of the child. This was also supported by attachment research as the maturation process is dependent on a good enough and facilitating environment (Winnicott 1965). If health is associated with maturation, then immaturity can be seen as unhealthy for the psyche and is also seen as a threat to the individual and, within parenthood, a heavy burden for the child development (ibid.).

First, however, this is evident for the family system, but the professional caregivers too have an empathic and regulatory function, as the child who spends a lot of time outside the family also needs an emotional and facilitating environment in the field of professional education. A burdened child especially needs this help and Anna Ornstein has described it as a therapeutic milieu where the professional caregiver is being placed (seen from the perspective of attachment) "in the second row."

This approach changes the role of the therapist. Even though the importance of the therapeutic transference relationship is not questioned (especially for the hour-to-hour structural diagnosis), the timely influence of the environmental factors has to be accepted by the therapist so that the hours spent in the therapeutic room (under specific conditions tailored to the patient), portray only an important but small snapshot of the patient's life and represents "real life" that consists of daily conflicts, affectional overstimulation, and other adverse environmental factors. In 1940, Erikson also emphasized the fundamentally different importance of the parents in comparison to the therapeutic relationship.

This conceptual change modifies naturally the structure of the therapeutic relationship as well as the processual setting. At the end of the treatment, the parents should have gained a psychic maturation in order to continue the child's resumed healthy developmental – without therapeutic support. In the language of attachment research this would be described as the parents being adequately and age appropriately better able to "read" and address the attachment and affective needs of the child without being entangled with their own unresolved conflicts.

At the end of this book I would like to cite the opening lines of H.-P. Hartmann's book (2001) *Empathie und therapeutischer Dialog* in which he referred Anna and Paul Ornstein's contributions to the clinical work of psychoanalytic self psychology:

> "What can we do that our children will no longer be victims of prosecution?" This question was asked by a woman addressed to the Dutch advocate and brilliant writer Abel Herzberg who survived the concentration camp in Bergen-Belsen. Herzberg looked at the women in silence for a while. Then he answered, calm and convinced, "This question is asked wrong – it should be asked the following 'How can we raise our children so that they will not be in later life arsonists, hangman, and hangman's assistants?'"
>
> (p. 7)

During the course of her long life Anna Ornstein experienced countless meaningful self-selfobjects – encounters that helped her after surviving the Holocaust – accompanied for more than 70 years by her husband Paul who died in January 2017 – to develop her early childhood core self. Her life experiences have expanded her introspection but also her external perception. All this contributed to acknowledge the great importance of environmental factors not only in early life but also over the course of the life span. On the background of analytic self psychology she could explain that a large number of failures within the primary relationship dialogue influence the development of the nucleus self. The growing child is dependent on environmental factors – especially in early life – i.e., is dependent on the primary and secondary caregivers. It has to be a therapeutic concern that the parents identify with the suffering of the child in order to initiate and achieve a reorganization with the support of the therapist. Therefore the treatment must be conducted with great empathy in regards to the parents in order to "pick them up" where their own psychic development in aspects that are now of great importance for the child has stagnated.

All parents want to be good parents, however, some are hindered because of their own life conditions and struggle to maturely and consistently fulfill these parental tasks. Experience has shown that the sensitivity of the therapist is eagerly accepted (especially during infant-/toddler-mother-/parent therapy), transmitting this "gift" immediately to the child, so that the trans-generational transfer of empathic failure is stopped. Individuals who had the chance to experience empathy and have internalized these experiences are less prone to becoming "arsonists, hangman, and hangman's assistants." With her concept from environmental centered analytic family therapy of a child who suffers, Anna Ornstein has developed an outstanding and realistic treatment form. This treatment form enables the child who suffers from environmentally difficult circumstances and their affected parents to develop the possibility of a therapeutic dialogue that helps to master developmental tasks and therefore facilitates maturation.

References

Erikson, E.H. (1940): Studies in the interpretation of play. *Genetic Psychol. Monogr.* 22, S. 557–671.

Ornstein, A.; Ornstein, P. (2001): *Empathie und Therapeutischer Dialog. Beiträge zur klinischen Praxis der psychoanalytischen Selbstpsychologie.* Ed. by H.-P. Hartmann, Gießen (Psychosozial).

Winnicott, D.N. (1965): *Maturational Processes and the Facilitating Environment.* London (Hogarth Press).

Permissions

Chapter 4: Ornstein, A. (1976): Making Contact with the Inner World of Child: Towards a Theory of Psychoanalytic Psychotherapy with Children. *Comprehensive Psychiatry* 17: Gruene and Stratton, New York. Elsevier, Amsterdam.

Chapter 6: Ornstein, A. (1990): Anne and Vivienne: The Early Adolescence of Two Young Teenagers. Reviewed by Anna Ornstein: D. Schave/B. Schave: Early Adolescence and the Search for the Self: A Developmental Perspective (1989). In: *Contemporary Psychiatry*, Vol. 9, Nr. 3, September 1990, S. 183–188: Anne and Vivienne: The Early Adolescence of Two Young Teenagers.

Chapter 7 © 1999 From Changing Patterns in Parenting: Comments on the Origin and Consequences of Unmodified Grandiosity by Anna Ornstein, in Progress in Self Psychology, V. 15: Pluralism in Self Psychology, edited by Arnold I. Goldberg. Reproduced by permission of Taylor and Francis Group, LLC, a division of Informa plc.

Chapter 8 © 1993 From Little Hans. His Phobia and His Oedipus Complex by Anna Ornstein, in *Freud's Case Studies: Self-Psychological Perspectives*, edited by Barry Magid. Reproduced by permission of Taylor and Francis Group, LLC, a division of Informa plc.

Chapter 10 © from *Childhood Losses, Adult Memories* in Akhtar, S. (Ed.) (2012): The Mother and Her Child. Reproduced with permission of The Licensor through PLSclear.

Index

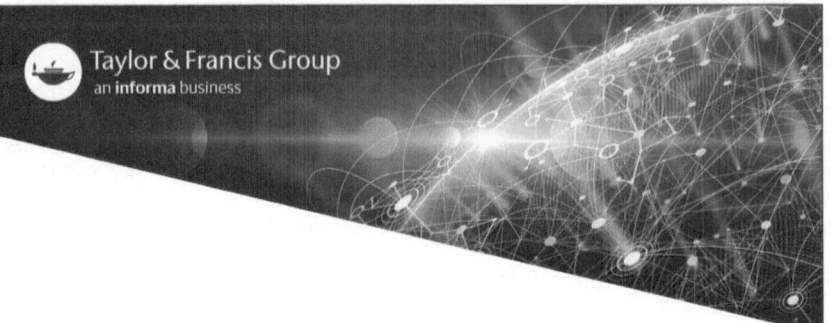

Taylor & Francis eBooks

www.taylorfrancis.com

A single destination for eBooks from Taylor & Francis
with increased functionality and an improved user
experience to meet the needs of our customers.

90,000+ eBooks of award-winning academic content in
Humanities, Social Science, Science, Technology, Engineering,
and Medical written by a global network of editors and authors.

TAYLOR & FRANCIS EBOOKS OFFERS:

A streamlined
experience for
our library
customers

A single point
of discovery
for all of our
eBook content

Improved
search and
discovery of
content at both
book and
chapter level

REQUEST A FREE TRIAL
support@taylorfrancis.com

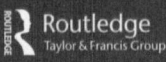 Routledge
Taylor & Francis Group

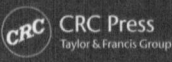 CRC Press
Taylor & Francis Group